ASTHMA

D1564345

LICENSE, DISCLAIMER OF LIABILITY, AND LIMITED WARRANTY

ASTHMA

David A. Olle

MERCURY LEARNING AND INFORMATION
Dulles, Virginia
Boston, Massachusetts
New Delhi

Publisher: David Pallai
MERCURY LEARNING AND INFORMATION
22841 Quicksilver Drive
Dulles, VA 20166
info@merclearning.com
www.merclearning.com
(800) 232-0223

3 1969 02563 0764

This book is printed on acid-free paper.

David A. Olle. *ASTHMA.*
ISBN: 978-1-683920-31-1

Library of Congress Control Number: 2017934663
171819 3 2 1

Printed in the United States of America

Our titles are available for adoption, license, or bulk purchase by institutions, corporations, etc.
For additional information, please contact the Customer Service Dept. at (800)232-0223(toll free).

All of our titles are available in digital format at authorcloudware.com and other digital vendors. *Companion files for this title are available by contacting info@merclearning.com.* The sole obligation of MERCURY LEARNING AND INFORMATION to the purchaser is to replace the book, based on defective materials or faulty workmanship, but not based on the operation or functionality of the product.

Table of Contents

PART TWO The Immune System as It Relates to Asthma and Allergies

CHAPTER 4 *How the Immune System Works*

CHAPTER 5 *The Inflammatory Immune Response*

PART THREE Diagnosis of Asthma

CHAPTER 6 *Seeing Your Doctor*

CHAPTER 10 *The EPR-3 Guidelines for Asthma Control*

CHAPTER 11 *Medications for Asthma*

Introduction

This book was inspired by recognition of the growing importance of asthma in the U.S. and around the world. Surprisingly, asthma incidence is increasing to a greater extent in the developed countries.

Asthma has a complex relationship with many other diseases and conditions which can present difficulties in the diagnosis of asthma, in monitoring the progression of the disease, and in the choices of treatments. When associated medical conditions are present, they can either aggravate asthma, or asthma can worsen the other conditions.

The book describes the basic principles of the respiratory system and how it relates to asthma. The immune system is described as a basis for understanding the relationship of asthma to allergies.

The methods used in the diagnosis and monitoring of asthma are presented as well as classification tables for asthma severity. The choices of asthma medications used are described in detail.

Practical applications that can be used by the asthma patient are essential features of this book. Topics include education, use of devices to administer medications, occupational hazards for the asthma patient, environmental factors in the home and outdoors, travel for the asthma patient, and special aspects of asthma for children and during pregnancy.

This book is designed to be a comprehensive background on asthma, and to encourage patients to be active participants in their own care. The accompanying Companion Files provide reference links for more information. As knowledge on asthma is continuously evolving, it is important to continue research on new methods of treatment and care.

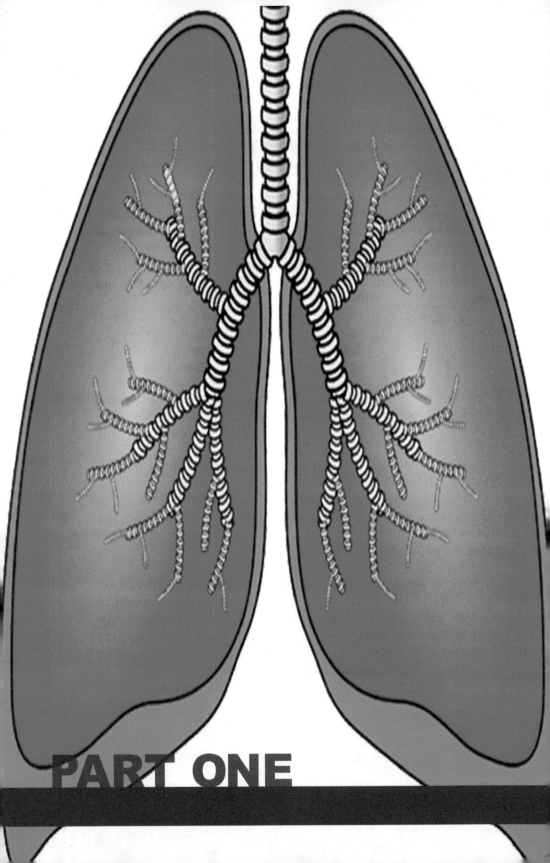

PART ONE

Introduction to Asthma

In Part One, we present a basic definition of asthma and its main symptoms. The normal respiratory system is described in some detail to provide a basis for understanding the changes taking place during the asthmatic condition. A brief introduction on the relationship of asthma to allergies is presented, along with theories on the roles of the microbiome and a clean environment during childhood on the development of asthma.

SOURCE: Medline Plus Magazine

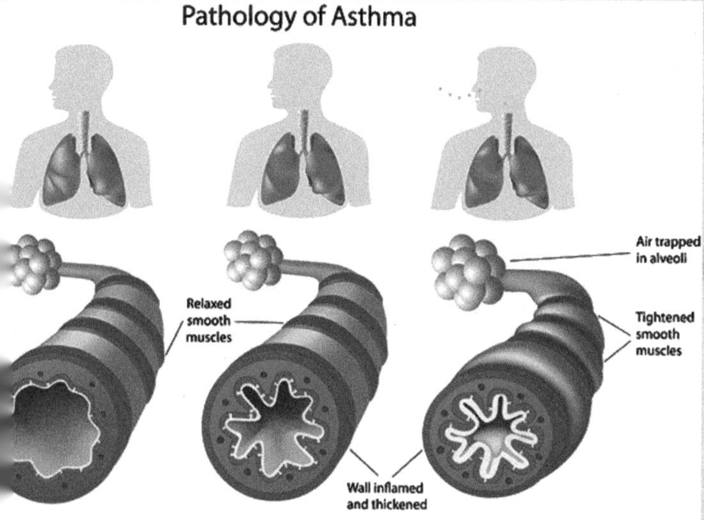

Pathology of Asthma

Air trapped in alveoli

Relaxed smooth muscles

Tightened smooth muscles

Wall inflamed and thickened

rmal airway

Asthmatic airway

Asthmatic airway during attack

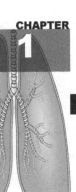

Fundamental concepts of asthma

1. What is asthma?

Asthma is a chronic (long-term) lung disease in which the airways become inflamed, narrow and swell, and produce extra mucus, which makes it difficult to breathe. Asthma is a very common disease and is increasing in importance. The disease commonly begins in childhood (although not always) and remains for a lifetime. The causes of asthma are complex but are thought to be a combination of the genetic makeup of the individual and the environment. Asthma is not a single disease but multiple diseases with similar clinical features.

A more comprehensive definition of asthma is presented in Question 34.

This figure illustrates the basic concepts of asthma:
- Asthma is a worldwide problem.
- Asthma affects twice as many boys than girls.

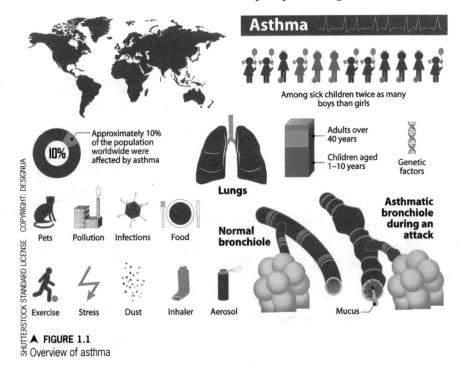

Asthma

Among sick children twice as many boys than girls

Approximately 10% of the population worldwide were affected by asthma

10%

Adults over 40 years

Children aged 1–10 years

Genetic factors

Lungs

Pets　Pollution　Infections　Food

Normal bronchiole

Asthmatic bronchiole during an attack

Exercise　Stress　Dust　Inhaler　Aerosol

Mucus

▲ FIGURE 1.1
Overview of asthma

- More children are affected by asthma than adults.
- Asthma affects the lungs; particularly the airway tubes known as the bronchi (singular- bronchiole).
- An asthma attack (exacerbation) involves swelling of the bronchi with the formation of mucus.
- Asthma can be caused by genetic factors or precipitated by environmental factors such as pets, pollution, infections, certain foods, exercise, stress, and dust.
- Common means of administering asthma medications include inhaler and aerosol.

2. What are the main symptoms of asthma?

The main symptoms of asthma are wheezing, cough, chest tightness, and shortness of breath. Symptoms of asthma can vary in intensity among individuals and within a given individual. Diagnosis of asthma can be difficult, but great strides have been made in recent years, resulting in physicians being able to treat successfully virtually all asthma cases. Modern asthma management is directed toward symptom prevention as well as symptom control. As we shall see, avoiding asthma triggers (substances that provoke asthma) is an important aspect of asthma prevention.

3. How prevalent is asthma?

Asthma is a very common disease found in all ages and ethnic groups, and its incidence continues to grow. The following summary is based on excellent reports issued by the U.S. Centers for Disease Control and Prevention (CDC).

 Prevalence is the percentage of the population having a condition at a specific point in time or during a given period, such as three months.

- The number of people with asthma continues to grow. One in 12 people (about 25 million, or 8% of the U.S. population) had asthma in 2009, compared with 1 in 14 (about 20 million, or 7%) in 2001.
- More than half (53%) of people with asthma had an asthma attack in 2008. More children (57%) than adults (51%) had an attack. In 2007, 185 children and 3,262 adults died from asthma.
- About 1 in 10 children (10%) had asthma, and 1 in 12 adults (8%) had asthma in 2009. women are compared to men, and boys compared to girls.

- In 2010, 3 out of 5 children who have asthma had one or more asthma attacks in the previous 12 months.
- For the period 2008–2010, asthma prevalence was higher among children than adults.
- In 2008 less than half of people with asthma reported being taught how to avoid triggers. Almost half (48%) of adults who were taught how to avoid triggers did not follow most of this advice.
- About 1 in 9 (11%) non-Hispanic blacks of all ages and about 1 in 6 (17%) of non-Hispanic black children had asthma in 2009, the highest rate among racial/ethnic groups.
- For the period 2008–2010, asthma prevalence was higher among multiple-race, black, and American Indian or Alaska Native persons than white persons.
- From 2001 through 2009, asthma rates rose the most among black children, almost a 50% increase.
- From 2001 through 2009, the greatest rise in asthma rates was among black children (almost a 50% increase).

The term "asthma attack" is falling out of favor with asthma professionals–the preferred name is now exacerbation.

Table 1.1 Asthma prevalence by selected demographic characteristics (2008–2010)

	Percent
Total prevalence	8.2
Children	9.5
Adults	7.7
Male	7.0
Female	9.2
White	7.7
Black	11.2
Hispanic	6.5
Living below poverty level	11.2

Although asthma has been increasing in the U.S., statistics suggest that asthma is better controlled in patients with asthma.

- In 2008, asthma hospitalizations were 1.5 times higher among female than male patients.
- From 2001 to 2009, health care visits for asthma per 100 persons with asthma declined in primary care settings, while asthma emergency department visit and hospitalization rates were stable.
- For the period 2007–2009, black persons had higher rates of asthma emergency department visits and hospitalizations per 100 persons with asthma than white persons and a higher asthma death rate per 1,000 persons with asthma. Compared with adults, children with asthma had more visits to primary care and emergency departments, similar hospitalization rates, and lower death rates.
- The cost of asthma is significant for the individual and society as a whole. In 2007, 185 children and 3,262 adults died from asthma. Asthma cost the US about $3,300 per person with asthma each year from 2002 to 2007 in medical expenses, missed school and work days, and early deaths.
- Asthma costs in the US grew from about $53 billion in 2002 to about $56 billion in 2007, about a 6% increase.
- More than half (59%) of children and one-third (33%) of adults who had an exacerbation missed school or work because of asthma in 2008. On average, in 2008 children missed four days of school and adults missed five days of work because of asthma.
- About 40% of uninsured people with asthma could not afford their prescription medicines, and about 11% of insured persons could not afford their medicines.

4. How do the lungs work?

The following is a discussion of the anatomical features of the normal respiratory system that are important in understanding the changes taking place during the asthmatic condition.

The respiratory system is made up of organs and tissues that help you breathe by taking up oxygen from the air and expelling carbon dioxide from the body.

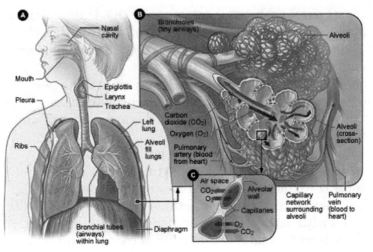

▲ FIGURE 1.2

Figure A shows the location of the respiratory structures in the body. Figure B is an enlarged view of the airways, alveoli (air sacs), and capillaries (tiny blood vessels). Figure C is a closeup view of gas exchange between the capillaries and alveoli. CO_2 is carbon dioxide, and O_2 is oxygen.
National Heart, Lung, and Blood Institute
http://www.nhlbi.nih.gov/health/health-topics/topics/hlw/system

When you breathe, air is taken up by the nose and passes through the nasal passages to the back of the throat. If you breathe through the mouth, air directly enters the throat. From the throat, the air continues until the larynx. The larynx is known as the voice box and consists of a cartilage skeleton housing the vocal cords. The larynx is covered by a flap of cartilage called the epiglottis. During breathing, the epiglottis is open, allowing air to pass into the trachea. The trachea or windpipe is a tube that connects the throat to the lungs. The trachea branches into two bronchial tubes which enter the lungs. Within the lungs, the bronchi continue to branch into successively narrower bronchi until they end in the smallest airway called the bronchiole. Each bronchiole leads into the air sacs, called alveoli. The alveoli are completely encircled by a network of tiny blood vessels called capillaries. Within the alveoli, gas exchange takes place. Oxygen is absorbed into the bloodstream by the capillaries, and waste carbon dioxide produced by the body is carried by the bloodstream to the capillary membranes, transferred to the alveoli, and exhaled by the lungs.

The main bronchi have relatively large lumens (internal cavities) that are lined by epithelium. Under the epithelium is a smooth muscle layer arranged as two ribbons of muscle that spiral in opposite directions. This smooth muscle layer contains seromucous glands, which secrete mucus. Bronchial smooth muscle contraction causes airway narrowing, thereby playing a role in asthma.

The transport of gases involved in respiration is carried out by pulmonary arteries and veins. The pulmonary artery carries deoxygenated blood from the heart to the lungs. As the pulmonary artery enters the lungs, it branches into successively smaller sizes until it becomes part of the capillary network. The blood in the capillaries is oxygenated and returns to the heart via the pulmonary veins.

The functioning of the lungs, and in particular the bronchi, is under control of the autonomic nervous system. This system consists of two branches: the sympathetic and parasympathetic branches. The resting bronchial smooth muscle tone is largely under the control of the parasympathetic nerves. Parasympathetic nerves are largely cholinergic, meaning that acetylcholine is used for transmission of the nerve impulse or stimulation of nerve receptors. Stimulation of cholinergic nerves causes constriction of the bronchi, mucus secretion, and bronchial vasodilation. As we shall see, constriction of the bronchi can be exaggerated during an exacerbation of asthma. Stimulating the sympathetic system has the opposite effect, namely the relaxation of the bronchial tubes. The sympathetic system is largely adrenergic, being stimulated by norepinephrine. These terms are important in understanding the action of asthma medications.

ON THE WEB

For an excellent animated discussion of the anatomy and physiology of the lungs and trachea, visit: https://www.youtube.com/watch?v=cR0_rJpkv8w

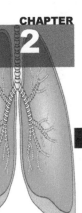

What factors influence the development of asthma?

5. What causes asthma?

The exact causes of asthma are still not known with certainty. Researchers believe genetic and environmental factors interact to cause asthma, most often early in life. These factors include:

Asthma is believed to be the result of a complex interaction between a person's genetic makeup and exposure to various environmental factors.

- An inherited tendency to develop allergies, called atopy.
- Parents who have asthma.
- Abnormal development and growth of the lungs during infancy.
- Certain respiratory infections during childhood.
- Contact with some airborne allergens or exposure to some viral infections in infancy or early childhood when the immune system is developing.
- Children and adults with asthma have an immune system that responds differently from those who do not have asthma.

Atopy is a genetic tendency to develop allergic diseases. Atopy is typically associated with heightened immune responses to common allergens.

If asthma or atopy runs in your family, exposure to irritants (e.g., tobacco smoke) may make your airways more reactive to substances in the air.

An allergen is a type of antigen that causes an inappropriate immune response known as an allergy. Allergens can enter the body by being inhaled, swallowed, touched or injected.

Some factors may be more likely to cause asthma in some people than in others. Researchers continue to explore what causes asthma.

The DNA molecule depicted in this diagram (in schematic form) is shown as a double helix held together by chemical bonds. The colored bars shown bonded together are chemical structures known as nucleotides. Genes exist as small sections of the DNA molecule.

Genes are the basic unit of inheritance which determines the particular characteristics or traits of a person. Genes exist as small sections of the DNA molecule which are located in the nucleus of the cell.

Asthma and allergic diseases are believed to be caused by multiple interacting genes, some having a protective effect and others contributing to the disease process, with each gene having its own tendency to be influenced by the environment. It is likely that the risk of developing asthma is greatest when both genetic and environmental risk factors are present simultaneously. More than 100 candidate genes have been identified to have an

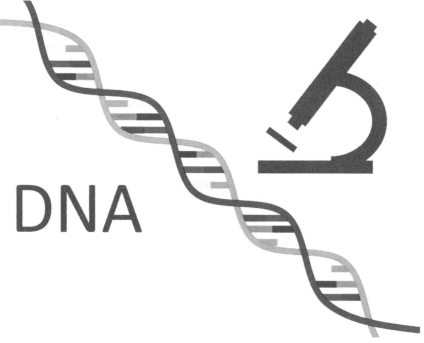

▲ Figure 2.1
DNA molecule
Source: Tumisu/Creative Commons
https://pixabay.com/p-1020670/?no_redirect

association with asthma. Current asthma research is focused on the involvement of genes in protecting the integrity of the bronchial epithelium, recognition of antigens or allergens, regulation of the immune system, and in the progression of asthma in the airway.

7. How does the immune system influence the asthmatic condition?

The immune system has an essential role in protecting the body against pathogenic organisms such as bacteria, viruses, and parasites. In doing so, the immune system must distinguish foreign material from the person's normal cells and tissues. The immune system has two main divisions. The innate or natural immune system is acquired at birth and provides an immediate but non-specific response to foreign material. The adaptive immune system, also known as acquired immunity, provides improved recognition of the pathogen and a form of immunological memory to launch more rapid and effective responses to subsequent encounters with the pathogen. The innate and immune systems work together to mount an effective immune response and are important in allergic responses as well. The immune system will be discussed in detail in Part Two.

An antigen is a protein or carbohydrate substance the immune system perceives as being foreign or dangerous. Antigens may be present on bacteria, viruses, tissue cells, or toxins and induce a specific immune response by the body.

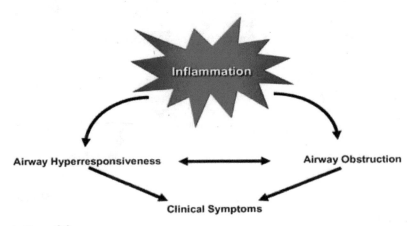

▲ Figure 2.2
Source: National Asthma Education and Prevention Program, Third Expert Panel on the Diagnosis and Management of Asthma.

The interplay and interaction between airway inflammation and the clinical symptoms and pathophysiology of asthma inflammation is now considered to play an overarching role in asthma. This figure illustrates how inflammation affects the airway to cause symptoms of asthma.

8. How does airway obstruction develop in asthma?

Airflow limitation in asthma continually recurs and is caused by a variety of changes in the airway. These include:

Bronchoconstriction. In asthma, the dominant physiological event leading to clinical symptoms is airway narrowing and a subsequent interference with airflow. In acute exacerbations of asthma, bronchial smooth muscle contraction (bronchoconstriction) occurs quickly to narrow the airways in response to exposure to a variety of stimuli including allergens or irritants. These stimuli cause bronchoconstriction by the release of chemical mediators from mast cells lining the bronchi. These chemicals include histamine, tryptase, leukotrienes, and prostaglandins. Aspirin and other nonsteroidal anti-inflammatory drugs can also cause acute airflow obstruction in some patients, and evidence indicates that this response also involves mediator release from airway cells. Also, other stimuli (including exercise, cold air, and irritants) can cause acute airflow obstruction. The mechanisms regulating the airway response to these factors are less well defined, but the intensity of the response appears related to underlying airway inflammation. Stress may also play a role in precipitating asthma exacerbations. Stress may cause increased generation of chemical mediators known as cytokines that promote inflammation.

Airway hyperresponsiveness. Airway hyperresponsiveness— an exaggerated bronchoconstrictor response to a wide variety of stimuli—is a major, but not necessarily unique feature of asthma. The mechanisms influencing airway hyperresponsiveness are multiple and include inflammation, dysfunctional regulation of nerves, and structural changes. Inflammation appears to be a major factor in determining the degree of airway hyperresponsiveness. Treatment directed toward reducing inflammation can reduce airway hyperresponsiveness and improve asthma control.

Airway obstruction. Chronic inflammation can result in the appearance of other factors that limit airflow. Increased airway obstruction can be due to swelling of the epithelial lining (edema), mucus hypersecretion and the formation of mucus plugs.

Airway remodeling refers to changes in the normal composition and structural organization of the bronchial tissue. Airway remodeling is a hallmark of chronic asthma that leads to permanent damage to the tissues. When these changes occur, asthma can be more difficult to treat. Although inflammation continues to be considered the driving force behind asthma, it is now believed that functionally active structural components are also involved. The bronchial epithelium provides a barrier that protects the lung against external environmental factors. When the epithelium is damaged or defective, pathogens and toxins can enter the bronchial tissue resulting in many detrimental changes, including fibrosis, increased mucus secretion, and increased smooth muscle mass. Rather than being a primary cause of asthma, allergen sensitization may well be the consequence of a defective airway epithelium. Injury to the epithelium activates production of immune cells that promote inflammation and fibrosis instead of repairing the injured tissue. Asthmatic airways are very susceptible to respiratory viruses and the impact of air pollutants on asthma exacerbations. Details of the immune system response will be discussed in Part Two.

> For a comprehensive discussion of remodeling in asthma, together with **ON THE WEB** excellent illustrations, visit: http://www.jacionline.org/article/S0091-6749(11)00748-2/pdf

9. What is the relationship of allergies to asthma?

Asthma and allergies are separate medical conditions, and it is common for a person to have both asthma and allergies simultaneously. An allergy is an immune system response to a substance known as an allergen resulting in physical symptoms. Asthma is a disease affecting the lungs with symptoms appearing as a result of certain triggers. A trigger is a stimulus to the development of asthma symptoms. An allergen does not cause asthma but is one of several triggers. A person can have asthma but not allergies. Children with coexisting allergic conditions (hay fever, food allergy, and eczema) are at greater risk of severe asthma.

A delayed immune response, also known as a cell-mediated response, results from the first exposure to an antigen. An immediate immune response results from reaction with antibodies (particularly IgE) in the blood. These antibodies were formed as a result of exposure to an antigen.

Secretion of histamine is an important part of the acute immune response of the body. Histamine secretion results in many of the symptoms of allergy, particularly allergic rhinitis, but to a lesser degree in asthma. Mast cells are located in the epithelial inner lining of the bronchi. Previous exposure to an allergen (antigen) causes an immune response resulting in the attachment of immune cells known as immunoglobin E (IgE) to the surface

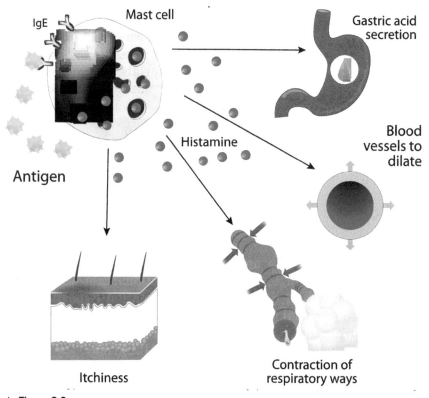

▲ **Figure 2.3**
Role of histamine in the asthmatic response
SOURCE: Shutterstock ID: 366310967
Copyright-Designa

The release of histamine from the mast cells results in many of the symptoms of allergy and asthma, including nasal itch and sneezing, runny nose and watery eyes, breathing difficulty (airway narrowing), and mucus secretion.

of mast cells. When allergen particles reenter the bronchi, they bind to IgE causing the release of histamine. As shown in the illustration, histamine causes contraction of the bronchi, dilation of blood vessels, and "itchiness" which in the case of asthma involves increased irritability and responsiveness of the bronchi to allergens. Histamine can also provoke mucus secretion and sneezing.

CASE STUDY

Jane was affected by asthma since early childhood. It was most likely hereditary as many of her family members also had asthma. The family had a beach house, and Jane experienced marked episodes of sneezing during their stays at the beach.

Eventually, the family determined that it was mold forming on the bed sheets, pillows, and blankets that caused Jane's allergy. For all subsequent visits, all these materials were thoroughly cleaned and covered, resulting in a marked reduction in asthmatic symptoms.

11. What is the difference between allergic and non-allergic asthma?

Allergic asthma is an immune response to allergens resulting in asthma symptoms. Allergic asthma typically begins in childhood. Most cases of allergic asthma are due to allergens that are inhaled.

Non-allergic asthma is more likely to be seen in adulthood. Non-allergic asthma is caused by infections that target the bronchial epithelium resulting in inflammation (Question 11), or by substances that irritate and damage the airways but not resulting in an immune response (Question 10). Non-allergic asthma has the reputation of being difficult to treat.

12. What are the primary allergens that can trigger allergic asthma?

• Dust mites found in bedding, clothing, and fabrics.

Both the body parts and feces of dust mites can act as allergens.

- Cockroaches are very widespread. The feces, body parts and saliva of cockroaches can serve as allergens.
- Sensitivity to sulfites, food additives, or aspirin.
- Molds that grow in places where moisture is present, both indoors and outdoors. Molds produce tiny spores which become airborne and are then inhaled.
- Dogs and cats produce allergens from their hair, saliva, feces, and urine.
- Pollen from trees, grasses, and weeds that become airborne are a common allergen. Specific pollens can peak in quantity at a certain season of the year.

13. What are the major irritants that can trigger non-allergic asthma?

- Smoke from tobacco, cooking, wood burning stoves, and fireplaces
- Fumes from unvented oil or gas stoves
- Household cleaners and air-freshening sprays
- Outside air pollution from ozone and airborne particles
- Building and paint products
- Cosmetics, perfumes, and hair sprays

14. What medical conditions can trigger non-allergic asthma?

- Common cold
- Sinusitis
- Influenza (flu)
- Gastroesophageal reflux disease (GERD)
- Bronchitis

15. What is the hygiene hypothesis?

The hygiene hypothesis arose from observational studies showing that people of industrialized countries appear to be more prone to asthma and allergies than those of undeveloped countries. The hypothesis proposes that adequate early childhood exposure to pathogens stimulates the proper development of the immune system. Under this proposal, a lack of exposure to harmful bacteria, viruses, and parasites during early childhood could result in an immature immune system that may not be able to distinguish between pathogenic organisms and innocuous substances. As a result, the immune system may launch an attack on a normally innocuous substance as if it were an invading organism.

The hygiene hypothesis initially focused on the effect of overuse of antibacterials and antibiotics, and where and how children are raised. Currently, more focus is shown on the influence of the microbial colonies inhabiting the body on the development of allergies (Question 16).

16. Does the microbiome have a relationship to asthma?

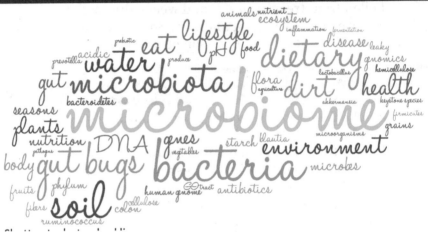

▲ **Figure 2.4**
Microbiome word cloud showing that many factors affect the microbiome
Shutterstock standard license
Copyright: arloo

The human microbiota consists of the microbial cells harbored by each person, while the human microbiome consists of the genes these cells harbor. The microbiota is found largely in the gastrointestinal tract (the gut) but also exists in the skin and respiratory tract. The microbiome consists largely of bacteria, but also includes viruses, protozoa, and fungi. The microbes constituting the microbiota have a symbiotic relationship with the host (our body), meaning that they both benefit. Before technology advances in gene analyses (sequencing), it was very difficult to study a person's microbiome. Previously, microbes could only be identified from laboratory cultures, a difficult and

A healthy microbial population in the body performs many vital functions and is essential for a person's well-being.

sometimes impossible task for some species.

The microbiome is now a very hot research topic with a rapidly evolving understanding of its functioning. The study of the microbiome was given a greater emphasis by the establishment of the federal Human Microbiome Project. Each person has a unique composition of gut microbes, although a core set of microbes is common to all people. The effect of the microbiome on the body's functioning turns out to be so wide-ranging that it is sometimes considered to be the "forgotten organ" (see Figure 2.3).

Research has shown that the microbiome may affect the following body functions:

- Allow digestion of otherwise indigestible carbohydrates
- Metabolic disorders associated with obesity and Type 2 diabetes
- Chronic liver diseases
- Inflammatory bowel diseases
- Colorectal cancer
- Allergies

To fully appreciate the importance of the microbiome, it is necessary to understand the interactions between the components of the microbiome and its host. Over the millennia, the association between the immune system and the microbiome have evolved to such an extent that the immune system requires interaction with the microbes for their proper development. The microbiota sends critical signals that promote the full development of immune cells and tissues, leading to protection from infections by pathogens. Critical in this association is the ability of the immune system to recognize the resident microbes as harmless.

The microbiome has been shown to have a profound effect on health or disease of the human host. The concept has arisen of a normal healthy microbiome in the gut that develops in the early life of the infant. Many factors can influence the development of the microbiome of the infant, including exposure of the mother to microbes before birth, gestational age, mode of delivery (cesarean or vaginal), genetics of the mother, and breastfeeding, while antibiotics and diet may also influence the microbiomes of older people. Many environmental factors can lead to disruption of the microbiome to the detriment of the host. Environmental factors such as the type of diet and the use of antibiotics in the infant can affect the gut microbiome and can be related to occurrences of asthma and allergies. Studies have shown that an altered diversity of gut microbiota during infancy as well as colonization with specific pathogenic bacteria has been linked with an elevated risk of allergy. Babies that had low or undetectable levels of four bacteria at three months old all went on to show early signs of asthma—wheezing and skin allergies—at a year old. Long-term use of antibiotics in adults results in a less diverse microbial population in the gut as well as changes in microbial species.

The presence of specific microbes serves as a stimulus to educate and mature the immune system. Studies have shown that certain microbes stimulate the formation of immune cells called regulatory T cells that suppress a hypersensitive immune system. Work is underway to characterize the microbiota of individuals with allergies.

Studies have shown an association between bronchial infections (including asthma) and the colonization of certain organisms in the bronchi. Other studies have focused on the role of the gut microbiome on asthma development. Epidemiological studies show that there are fewer cases of childhood asthma among children who are exposed to microbial rich environments, such as the presence of livestock and pets or other siblings. Exposure to microbes aids development of the immune system, while movement of immune cells by the blood to the respiratory tract can influence asthma development as well.

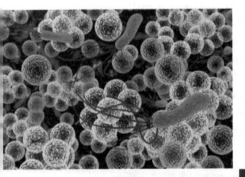

▲ Figure 2.5
The healthy microbiome consists of many beneficial microbial species
SOURCE: National Institute of Environmental Health Sciences, National Institutes of Health. This image is from a podcast presented on March 2, 2015 by the sponsorship of Partnership for Environmental Public Health.
https://www.niehs.nih.gov/research/supported/translational/peph/podcasts/microbiome/index.cfm

17. How is asthma currently viewed?

Traditionally, the basic cause of asthma was thought to be due to airway constriction caused by tightening of the muscles surrounding the bronchial tubes. It is now understood that airway constriction is due to inflammation.

What conditions are related to asthma?

CHAPTER 3

18. How are pneumonia infections associated with asthma?

Pneumonia and asthma both affect the lungs. Two pneumonia-causing bacteria species that appear to be associated with asthma are *Mycoplasma pneumoniae* and *Chlamydia pneumoniae*. *M. pneumoniae* infections can precede the onset of asthma, exacerbate asthmatic symptoms, and cause difficulties with asthma management. Although an association between *M. pneumoniae* infections and asthma has been known for more than two decades, the nature of the association is still not clear. Pneumonia infections may stimulate immune system components already existing in the asthma patient.

Acute C. pneumoniae infection can cause exacerbation of asthma, and chronic or persistent infection has been linked to chronic or persistent asthma and adult-onset asthma. Persistent or recurring infection with *C. pneumoniae* may amplify asthmatic inflammation.

There are many medical conditions that produce symptoms similar to asthma. Some conditions are extensions of asthma and allergies, and sometimes asthma can aggravate symptoms of related diseases. Some conditions have symptoms that mimic asthma without being asthma at all. Although it is often popularly thought that related conditions bring about asthma, it is more likely that they act by aggravating a pre-existing asthma condition. Various parts of the respiratory system are united by a common mucosal layer and interconnected nerves. The common symptoms observed by the different conditions can be related to this united system.

19. What is allergic rhinitis?

Rhinitis is inflammation of the nasal mucus membranes. Rhinitis is classified into three types: (1) infectious rhinitis due to bacterial or virus infections, including the common cold, (2) nonallergic rhinitis, and (3) allergic rhinitis, the most common type of rhinitis.

Allergic rhinitis is commonly known as hay fever, a form of allergy. Allergic rhinitis typically affects the nose, which can be runny or stuffy, accompanied with sneezing. Complications of hay fever include infections of the eyes, middle ear, and sinuses.

Although allergic rhinitis affects the upper airways, and asthma is a condition of the lower airways, they often exist together and share key elements of pathogenesis. Some researchers even consider asthma and allergic rhinitis to be manifestations of the same disease, as the nasal and bronchial mucosas are elements of a "united airway." Patients with allergic rhinitis and no clinical evidence of asthma commonly exhibit nonspecific bronchial hyperresponsiveness. Allergic rhinitis is itself a risk factor for the development of asthma and may exacerbate coexisting asthma. Allergic rhinitis may also confound the diagnosis of asthma.

Several possibilities have been proposed to link involvement of the nose and bronchi, including:

- Inhalation of postnasal drip containing inflammatory cells and proinflammatory (capable of stimulating inflammation) cells into the lungs
- A neural reflex involving the nose and pharynx
- An increased exposure of the lower airways to dry and cold air. This increased exposure is due to increased mouth breathing caused by nasal obstruction

Treatment of chronic rhinitis not only reduces nasal inflammation obstruction and discharge but also can reduce lower airway hyperresponsiveness and symptoms of asthma.

20. What is COPD?

COPD is short for chronic obstructive pulmonary disease. Although some of the symptoms of persons with COPD may resemble asthma, such as coughing and wheezing, the causes are different. Cigarette smoking is the leading cause of COPD, although long-term exposure to pollution can also be a contributing factor. Most people who have COPD have both emphysema and chronic bronchitis. In emphysema, the air sacs in the lungs lose their elasticity resulting in a reduction of gas exchange in the lungs (see lung anatomy in Question 5). In chronic bronchitis, the lining of the airways is constantly irritated and inflamed causing the lining to thicken. A lot of thick mucus forms in the airways, making it hard to breathe.

It is important for the physician to distinguish between COPD and asthma. The medications used in the two diseases are different, and asthma patients have a better chance of recovery.

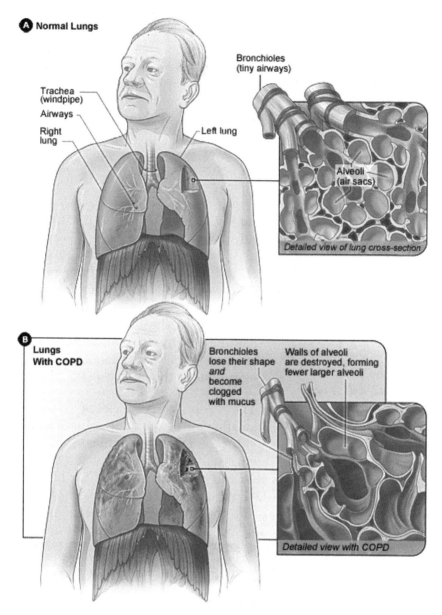

A Normal Lungs

Trachea
(windpipe)

Airways

Right
lung

Left lung

Bronchioles
(tiny airways)

Alveoli
(air sacs)

Detailed view of lung cross-section

B Lungs
With COPD

Bronchioles
lose their shape
and
become
clogged
with mucus

Walls of alveoli
are destroyed, forming
fewer larger alveoli

Detailed view with COPD

▲ Figure 3.1
Normal lungs and lungs with COPD
Source: National Heart, Lung, and Blood Institute

21. What is GERD?

GERD is short for gastroesophageal reflux disease. GERD is commonly known as acid reflux and occurs when stomach contents flow back into the esophagus. GERD occurs when the lower esophageal sphincter valve separating the stomach from the esophagus does not function properly. After eating large meals, there is a buildup of gases in the stomach. These gases are released by burping or belching, causing a relaxation of the sphincter valve and entry of gas and stomach contents into the esophagus. This process is known as regurgitation.

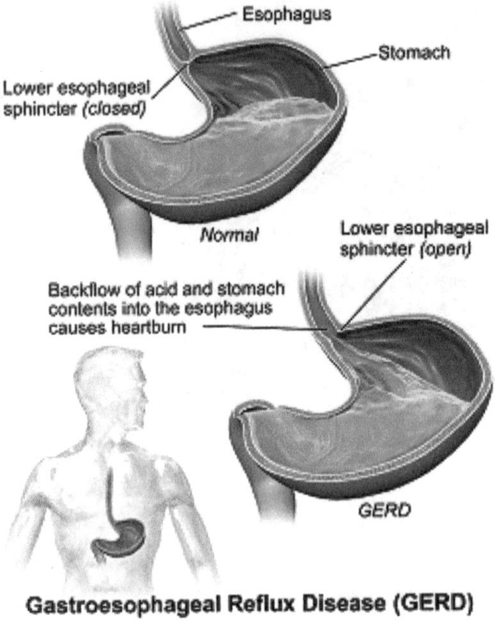

GERD is related to asthma through the process of aspiration, which is the drawing up of microdroplets of refluxate into the pharynx and trachea. These microdroplets contain acid and bile which are very irritating to the bronchi, potentially leading to chronic cough, laryngitis, and aspiration pneumonia, as well as aggravating the symptoms of allergy.

The epiglottis closes during swallowing to allow the bolus of food to enter the esophagus while prohibiting entry of food into the trachea. During breathing, the epiglottis opens to allow air to enter the trachea. During aspiration, stomach gases may go up the esophagus, pass through the epiglottis, and into the trachea.

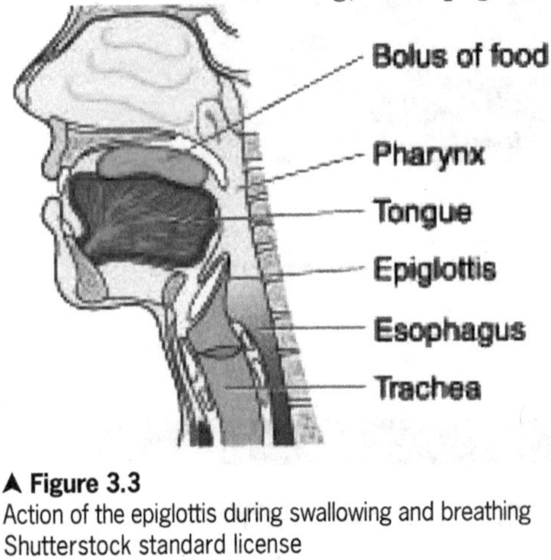

Gastroesophageal Reflux Disease (GERD)

▲ Figure 3.2

Gastrointestinal tract of normal and GERD persons
Source: https://commons.wikimedia.org/wiki/File:
GERD.png
"GERD.png" Licensed under Creative Commons
Attribution-Share Alike 4.0 International.

▲ Figure 3.3

Action of the epiglottis during swallowing and breathing
Shutterstock standard license
Copyright: Blamb

22. How are respiratory viral infections related to asthma?

Viral respiratory infections have been estimated to account for more than 80% of acute exacerbations of asthma in children and at least 30% to 40% of exacerbations in adults with asthma. The most significant asthma-associated viruses include respiratory syncytial virus (RSV) and rhinovirus. Influenza, parainfluenza, and coronaviruses are less often associated with asthma. Viral infections are more important than bacterial infection for causing exacerbations.

The interaction of respiratory virus infection and chronic asthmatic airway inflammation results in respiratory symptoms that are more severe than those suffered by non-asthmatic persons. Whether respiratory viruses cause subsequent asthma is unclear. Several theories have been considered to account for the role of virus infections on asthma exacerbations. Exacerbation may occur because of an interaction between viral and asthmatic pathologies, or by sharing the 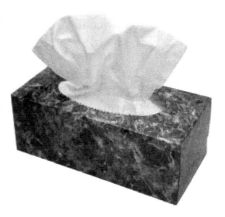 same disease mechanism in an additive manner. Virus infection might increase the sensitivity of the asthmatic airway to triggers such as allergen exposure.

Human rhinoviruses are the most frequent cause of the common cold and account for about 50% of virus-induced asthma exacerbations. Rhinoviruses are common in all age groups. Although rhinoviruses normally establish in the upper airway, there is convincing evidence that they can reproduce in the lower airway as well. This fact strengthens the role of rhinoviruses in causing exacerbations of asthma. Infants who develop virus-induced wheezing episodes are at increased risk for asthma if the infant is predisposed to develop asthma. How can colds lead to exacerbations of asthma? The inflammatory cells generated during colds could be aspirated into the lungs. There could be a neural reflex involving the nose and bronchi that could lead to bronchospasm. The viral infection stimulates the production of immune cells that cause inflammation. It has been proposed that a damaged airway epithelium could cause asthma exacerbations upon exposure to rhinovirus. The epithelium could be damaged by inflammatory cells from an allergy, or from air pollutants that have a direct toxic effect on the cells. The damaged epithelium can expose sensory nerves, which increases stimulation of sensory nerves by inhaled particles or inflammatory mediators.

Respiratory syncytial virus (RSV) is very common in young children, affecting almost 100% by age 3. RSV causes a severe bronchiolitis (inflammation of the bronchi) which is frequently associated with recurring wheezing and asthma. It is not clear if RSV accelerates the onset of asthma, or if the virus is involved in the allergic sensitization characteristic of asthma.

Parainfluenza viruses are very common and cause upper respiratory infections such as colds, bronchitis, and pneumonia. Despite the name, parainfluenza viruses are different viruses than flu viruses.

The Centers for Disease Control and Prevention (CDC) recommend receiving an annual seasonal influenza vaccine for all persons aged six months and older. Despite mixed evidence of whether vaccination prevents influenza-related asthma exacerbations in asthmatics, there are no better present options to prevent influenza. If one does not contract influenza, one cannot develop influenza-related asthma exacerbations, and therefore vaccination is still strongly favored by expert opinion.

Coronaviruses are another cause of infection of the nose, sinuses, and upper throat. Although most coronavirus infections are not serious, if the infection spreads to the lungs it can cause pneumonia and severe acute respiratory syndrome (SARS). The involvement of coronaviruses in asthma exacerbations has been recently revealed by the latest molecular methods, although coronavirus is not considered a major cause of exacerbations.

23. Are sinus disease and asthma related?

Disease of the nose and sinuses is the most common comorbidity associated with asthma. Rhinitis, sinusitis, and asthma may represent part of one disease process with manifestations at different sites. Patients with nasal symptoms appear to experience poorer asthma control.

Active sinusitis can aggravate asthma based on several possibilities:

Sinuses are hollow cavities located in the bones of the skull and face. Sinuses are connected to the nasal passages by small tubes or channels. Sinuses and their passages are coated with mucus membranes.

- The sinuses and lungs share common nervous and epithelial tissues and respond together when one is threatened.

Sinusitis is inflammation of the sinuses.

- Postnasal drip may trigger cough and asthmatic inflammation.
- Exposure to environmental irritants, infections, and allergens affect the mucosal lining of the sinus and lower airway simultaneously.

24. Are food allergies and asthma related?

Food intolerance is by far the more common cause of food hypersensitivity than is allergy. Food intolerance is a reaction to a certain food, but the reaction may only happen when you eat a lot of the offending food or eat the food often. Food intolerance usually comes on gradually and is not life threatening.

Food hypersensitivity consists of food intolerance and food allergy. Food intolerance is a response of the digestive system resulting in an inability to break down the food eaten. The European Academy of Allergy and Clinical Immunology now considers the preferred term for food intolerance to be non-allergic food hypersensitivity. A food allergy involves the immune system and is a more serious condition.

Food intolerance can be caused by the following:

- The absence of an enzyme needed to digest a particular food fully. Lactose intolerance is a common example.
- Irritable bowel syndrome (IBS) is a motility (spontaneous movement) disorder of the digestive tract that can cause abdominal pain, constipation, and diarrhea. IBS is very common affecting up to 20% of the adult population. IBS primarily involves the colon, although some people have symptoms indicating the involvement of the upper gastrointestinal tract as well. The syndrome is poorly understood but may be due to abnormal contraction and relaxation of the muscles lining the gastrointestinal tract. Certain foods have been known to trigger symptoms of the syndrome. Although IBS affects the gastrointestinal tract, while asthma affects the respiratory tract, many studies have shown that the two conditions frequently occur together. The reasons for the association have been difficult to determine but may involve an underlying neuromuscular disorder.

- Food poisoning. Toxins such as bacteria in spoiled food can cause severe digestive symptoms.
- Sensitivity to food additives. Sulfites are the main culprit and can provoke acute and occasionally severe episodes of bronchoconstriction. Sulfites are commonly added to foods as well as used in medications for the treatment of allergic diseases and asthma. Although monosodium glutamate and the yellow dye tartrazine had been thought to provoke asthma, well-designed clinical studies have failed to show that these additives can cause bronchoconstriction.
- Stress may trigger allergic reactions in the gut and other organs, and depression or anxiety may worsen symptoms in inflammatory disorders of the intestine.
- Celiac disease is an autoimmune condition, where an immune response (inflammation) is directed against one's body rather than against foreign substances such as viruses or bacteria. Celiac disease can only develop in those with certain genes. This chronic digestive condition is triggered by eating gluten, a protein found in wheat and other grains. The immune system of a person with celiac disease reacts negatively to the presence of gluten in the diet causing damage to the inner lining of the small bowel which reduces the person's ability to absorb nutrients. Celiac disease affects about 1% of the population. Another condition called non-celiac gluten sensitivity (NCGS) can cause similar symptoms but is not considered an autoimmune disease. Although celiac disease and possibly NCGS affect the immune system, they are not allergic diseases since they do not stimulate the production of IgE antibodies, characteristic of allergic diseases. People with celiac disease are more likely to develop asthma than people without asthma, and those with asthma are more likely to develop celiac disease.

Food allergy, similar to other types of allergies, is due to an inappropriate immune response to the food.

Both food allergy and food intolerance can cause nausea, stomach pain, vomiting, and diarrhea. The two conditions can be distinguished by certain symptoms. Food intolerance can cause gas or bloating, heartburn, headaches, or irritability. Food allergy can cause rash, hives, or itchy skin; shortness of breath;

chest pain; or an exacerbation.

Many studies have shown an association of asthma with food allergies. However, it is important to note that, contrary to public perception, studies have not shown that food allergies can cause asthma. Asthmatic children have a higher frequency of food allergies than in the general population. Asthmatic patients have a greater risk of being sensitized to certain foods associated with food allergies. Several findings suggest that coexistence of asthma and food allergy increases the severity of each of the disorders. The presence of a food allergy is a risk factor for the future development of asthma.

Allergic sensitization to foods is linked to more severe asthma. Avoidance of specific foods or additives has not been shown to improve asthma, even in patients who may perceive that a particular food worsens their asthma. However, patients with underlying asthma are more likely to experience a fatal or near-fatal food reaction known as anaphylaxis.

 Anaphylaxis is an acute allergic reaction affecting many parts of the body (systemic) that is potentially fatal. People with asthma that is associated with allergies are at greater risk for more severe anaphylaxis symptoms.

When you come into contact with a food allergen, your immune system overreacts and releases a chemical called histamine. The release of histamine causes the symptoms of an allergic reaction. These symptoms can include red, itchy, watery eyes and nose, sneezing, a scratchy or sore throat and itchy skin. For anyone with a food allergy, symptoms can also include wheezing and coughing. In people who have asthma, it can also trigger asthma symptoms such as coughing, tightness in the chest and difficulty breathing.

Asthma might be triggered by foods, but this is rare. There is some evidence that if you have both asthma and a food allergy, you may be at greater risk of having an exacerbation that is life-threatening, so it is very important to avoid the food. The most common foods associated with allergic symptoms are:

Eggs
Milk

Peanuts
Tree nuts (cashews, almonds, filberts, etc.)
Soy
Wheat
Fish
Shellfish

Although also rare, food additives can also trigger asthma. These additives are used as preservatives in food processing or preparation, and can be found in the following foods:

Dried fruits or vegetables
Potatoes (packaged and some prepared)
Wine and beer
Bottled lime or lemon juice
Shrimp (fresh, frozen, or prepared)
Pickled foods

Examples of food additives that can cause adverse reactions are

1. Sulfites–used as preservatives to prevent foods from turning brown.
2. Aspartame (Nutrasweet)–a calorie-free sweetener used in foods and beverages.
3. Parabens–used to preserve foods and medications. Also used in sunscreens and shampoos.
4. Tartrazine–a yellow dye used in foods and beverages.
5. Monosodium glutamate (MSG)–used to enhance flavor in packaged meats and foods.
6. Nitrates and nitrites–used to preserve foods, prevent botulism infection, enhance flavors, and color foods.
7. BHT and BHA–preservative chemicals added to cereals.

25. How can exposure to pets trigger asthma?

Cats and dogs are potent triggers of allergic and asthmatic attacks. The allergens are found in the animals' dander (skin scales), saliva and urine. These allergens get on the skin when the animal licks itself, the substance dries and eventually the skin flakes off. An animal's fur can collect allergens present in pollen, dust, and mold, and spread the allergens throughout the house. These allergens cause inflammation.

26. How are gastrointestinal tract allergies related to asthma?

How might gastrointestinal tract symptoms such as abdominal pain, nausea, and vomiting be related to asthma? Studies have shown physiological and histological abnormalities of the gastrointestinal tract in patients with allergic disease. Children with allergic diseases such as asthma and atopic dermatitis experience increased gastrointestinal symptoms.

The following are examples of gastrointestinal tract allergies:
- Gastrointestinal anaphylaxis–a very severe systemic reaction that can be life-threatening.
- Allergic eosinophilic esophagitis–a rare condition characterized by swelling of the esophagus caused by massive infiltration of eosinophils. The disease may be related to asthma.
- Oral allergy syndrome–consists of itching and swelling of the lips, the oral mucosa, and the soft palate immediately after eating raw fruits or vegetables.

27. What are drug allergies?

Drug allergies refer to certain drugs that produce allergic reactions in susceptible persons. Drug allergies typically occur in young and middle-aged adults and are more common in women than men.

Drug hypersensitivities provoking allergy largely involve stimulating the immune system. Drugs can also directly stimulate the release or activation of inflammatory mediators.

Examples of drugs that can cause allergic reactions are
1. Penicillin is the most frequent drug allergy.
2. Sulfonamides.
3. Cephalosporins are broad spectrum antibiotics resembling penicillin.
4. Radiocontrast agents are a type of medical contrast medium used to improve pictures of the inside of the body produced by various radiological procedures.
5. Local anesthetics.
6. General anesthetics.
7. Aspirin/NSAIDs.

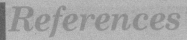

REFERENCES

References

CHAPTER 1

1. American Academy of Allergy, Asthma & Immunology. "Asthma statistics." 2016.
   http://www.aaaai.org/about-aaaai/newsroom/asthma-statistics

2. Centers for Disease Control and Prevention. "Asthma in the US," *Vital Signs*, May 2011.
   http://www.cdc.gov/VitalSigns/pdf/2011-05-vitalsigns.pdf

3. Lewis, M., A. Short & K. Lewis. "Autonomic nervous system control of the cardiovascular and respiratory systems in asthma." *Respiratory Medicine*. 100 (2006): 1688–1705.
   http://www.resmedjournal.com/article/S0954-6111(06)00050-3/pdf

4. National Center for Health Statistics. "Trends in asthma prevalence, health care use, and mortality in the United States, 2001–2010." 2012.
   http://www.cdc.gov/nchs/data/databriefs/db94.htm

5. National Heart, Lung, and Blood Institute. "What is ssthma?" Aug. 4, 2014. *https://www.nhlbi.nih.gov/health/health-topics/topics/asthma*

6. Van der Velden, V. and A. Hulsmann. "Autonomic innervation of human airways: structure, function, and pathophysiology in asthma." *Neuroimmunomodulation*. 6, (1999):145–159.
   http://www.karger.com/Article/Abstract/26376

CHAPTER 2

7. Asthma and Allergy Foundation of America. "Allergens and allergic asthma." Sept. 2015.
   http://www.aafa.org/page/allergic-asthma.aspx

8. Al-Muhsen, Jill Johnson, and Qutaybs Hamid. "Remodeling in asthma." *J Allergy Clin Immunol*. 128, no.3 (2011):451–462.
   http://www.jacionline.org/article/S0091-6749(11)00748-2/pdf

9. Bara, I., A. Ozier, J. Tunon de Lara, , R. Marthan, and P. Berger. "Pathophysiology of bronchial smooth muscle remodelling in asthma." *European Respiratory Journal*. 36, no. 5 (2010):1174–1184.
   http://erj.ersjournals.com/content/erj/36/5/1174.full.pdf

10. Bendoks, Meike and Matthias Kopp. "The relationship between advances in understanding the microbiome and the maturing hygiene hypothesis." *Current Allergy and Asthma Reports*. 13, no. 5 (2013):487–494.
    http://link.springer.com/article/10.1007%2Fs11882-013-0382-8

11. Bijanzadeh, Mahdi, , Padukudru A. Mahesh, and Nallur B. Ramachandra. "An understanding of the genetic basis of asthma." *Indian Journal of Medical Research*. 134, no. 2 (Aug. 2011):149–161.
    https://www.ncbi.nlm.nih.gov/pmc/articles/PMC3181014/

12. BioLegend. "Innate immunity resource guide." March 2008
    https://www.biolegend.com/media_assets/literature/images/InnateImmunityResourceGuide_3.pdf

13. Chow, Janet, S. Melanie Lee, Yue Shen, Arya Khosravi, and Sarkis K. Mazmanian. "Host-bacterial symbiosis in health and disease." *Adv Immunol*. 107 (2010):243–274.
    https://www.ncbi.nlm.nih.gov/pmc/articles/PMC3152488/pdf/nihms314235.pdf

14. Clemente, Jose, Luke K. Ursell, Laura Wegener Parfrey, and Rob Knight. "The impact of the gut microbiota on human health: an integrative view." *Cell.* 148 (2012):1258–1270.
   http://www.cell.com/cell/pdf/S0092-8674(12)00104-3.pdf

15. European Food Information Council. "The role of gut microorganisms in human health." *Food Today.* Oct. 2013.
   http://www.eufic.org/article/en/artid/The_role_of_gut_microorganisms_in_human_health/

16. Holgate, Stephen, Graham Roberts , Hasan S. Arshad , Peter H. Howarth , and Donna E. Davies. "The role of the airway epithelium and its interaction with environmental factors in asthma pathogenesis." *Proceedings of the American Thoracic Society.* 6 (2009):655–659.
   http://www.atsjournals.org/doi/abs/10.1513/pats.200907-072DP#readcube-epdf

17. Huang, Yvonne and Homer Boushey. "The microbiome in asthma." *J Allergy Clin Immunol.* 135, no. 1 (2015):25–30.
   http://www.ncbi.nlm.nih.gov/pmc/articles/PMC4287960/pdf/nihms645415.pdf

18. Meng, Jian-Feng and Lanny Rosenwasser. "Unraveling the genetic basis of asthma and allergic diseases." *Allergy Asthma Immunol Res.* 2, no.4 (2010): 215–227.
   https://www.ncbi.nlm.nih.gov/pmc/articles/PMC2946699/pdf/aair-2-215.pdf

19. New York Dept. of Health. "Environmental asthma triggers." No. 4955. 2006.
   https://www.health.ny.gov/publications/4955.pdf

20. Okada, C. Kuhn, H. Feillet and J. Bach. "The 'hygiene hypothesis' for autoimmune and allergic diseases: an update." *Clinical and Experimental Immunology.* 160, (2010):1–9.
   http://www.ncbi.nlm.nih.gov/pmc/articles/PMC2841828/pdf/cei0160-0001.pdf

21. Riiser, Amund. "The human microbiome, asthma, and allergy." *Allergy Asthma Clin Immunol BioMed Central* 11, no. 35 (2015).
   http://www.ncbi.nlm.nih.gov/pmc/articles/PMC4674907/pdf/13223_2015_Article_102.pdf

22. Romanet-Manent, S. Charpin, A. Magnan, A. Lanteaume, , D. Vervloet, and the EGEA Cooperative Group. "Allergic vs nonallergic asthma: what makes the difference?" *Allergy.* 57 (2002): 607–613.
   http://fmc.epneumo.fr/files/a7ac2de119748323860abb4081ed1229_1.pdf

23. Tinkelman, David. "Asthma: causes." *National Jewish Health.* April 1, 2012.
   https://www.nationaljewish.org/healthinfo/conditions/asthma/causes

24. Ursell, Luke, Jessica L Metcalf, Laura Wegener Parfrey, and Rob Knight. "Defining the human microbiome." *Nutrition Reviews.* 70, (Suppl 1): (Aug. 2012):S38–S44.
   https://www.ncbi.nlm.nih.gov/pmc/articles/PMC3426293/pdf/nihms369735.pdf

25. White, M. "The role of histamine in allergic diseases." *J Allergy Clin Immunol.* 86,no. 4 (Pt 2)(1990):599–605.
   https://www.ncbi.nlm.nih.gov/pubmed/1699987

26. Williams, Sarah. "Gut bacteria could predict asthma in kids." *Science News*. Sept. 30, 2015.
http://www.sciencemag.org/news/2015/09/gut-bacteria-could-predict-asthma-kids

27. Willyard, Cassandra. "Gut reaction." *Nature*. 479 (2011):S5–S7.
http://www.nature.com/nature/journal/v479/n7374_supp/pdf/479S5a.pdf

CHAPTER 3

28. American Academy of Allergy, Asthma & Immunology. "Influenza vaccination in asthmatic patients: is there benefit?" 2014.
https://www.aaaai.org/global/latest-research-summaries/Current-JACI-Research/influenza-vaccination-asthma

29. Buret, Andre. "How stress induces intestinal hypersensitivity." *Am J Pathol*. 168, no. 1 (2006):3–5.
https://www.ncbi.nlm.nih.gov/pmc/articles/PMC1592668/

30. Caffarelli, Carlo, Franca Maria Deriu, Vittorio Terzi, Francesca Perrone, Gianluigi dè Angelis, and David J Atherton. "Gastrointestinal symptoms in patients with asthma." *Arch Dis Child*. 82 (2000):131–135.
https://www.ncbi.nlm.nih.gov/pmc/articles/PMC1718218/pdf/v082p00131.pdf

31. Cafarelli, Carlo, M. Garrubba, C. Greco,C. Mastrorilli, and D. Povesi. "Asthma and food allergy in children: is there a connection or interaction?" *Frontiers in Pediatrics*. 4, no. 34 (2016):1–7.
https://www.ncbi.nlm.nih.gov/pubmed/27092299

32. Diaz, Gonzales and Arias Cruz. "Allergic rhinitis and asthma: 2 illnesses. The same disease?" *Rev Alerg* Mex 49, no. 1 (2002):20–24.
http://www.ncbi.nlm.nih.gov/pubmed/12070894

33. Dixon, Anne. "Rhinosinusitis and asthma: the missing link." *Curr Opin Pulm Med* 15, no. 1 (2009):19–24.
http://www.ncbi.nlm.nih.gov/pmc/articles/PMC2774711/pdf/nihms111084.pdf

34. Folkerts, Gert, Busse, W.,Nijkamp, F., Sorkness, R., and Gern, J. "Virus-induced airway hyperresponsiveness and asthma." *Am J Respir Crit Care Med*. 157 (1998):1708–1720.
http://www.atsjournals.org/doi/full/10.1164/ajrccm.157.6.9707163#.WAaCU-ArKc0

35. Gelfand, Erwin. "Respiratory viral infections and asthma: is there a link?" *Medscape*. 2000.
http://www.medscape.com/viewarticle/408755

36. Gern, James. "The ABCs of rhinoviruses, wheezing, and asthma." *J Virology*. 84, no. 15 (2010):7418–7426.
http://jvi.asm.org/content/84/15/7418.full.pdf

37. Gern, James. and William Busse. "Association of rhinovirus infections with asthma." *Clinical Microbiology Reviews*. 12, no.1 (1999):9–18.
https://www.ncbi.nlm.nih.gov/pmc/articles/PMC88904/pdf/cm000009.pdf

38. Hong, Soo-Jong. "The role of mycoplasma pneumoniae infection in asthma." *Allergy Asthma Immunol Res*. 4 (2012):59–61.
http://www.ncbi.nlm.nih.gov/pmc/articles/PMC3283794/pdf/aair-4-59.pdf

39. Kennedy, T., Jones, R., Hunginb, A., O'Flanagan, H., and Kelly, P. "Irritable bowel syndrome, gastro-oesophageal reflux, and bronchial hyper-responsiveness in the general population." *Gut*. 43 (1998): 770–774.
   http://gut.bmj.com/content/43/6/770.full.pdf+html?sid=30e43ef4-1142-4c30-9dcb-f62cfca352e0

40. Metcalfe, Dean. *Food allergy: adverse reactions to foods and food additives*, 4th edn. Blackwell Publishing, 2008.
   https://www.researchgate.net/profile/Julie_Nordlee/publication/230209029_Food_Allergy_Adverse_Reactions_to_Foods_and_Food_Additives_Fifth_Edition/links/02e7e5302a10aa3fda000000.pdf#page=347

41. Message, Simon and Sebastian Johnson. "Viruses in asthma: The role of viruses in childhood respiratory infections." *British Medical Bulletin*. 61, no. 1 (2002):29–43.
   http://bmb.oxfordjournals.org/content/61/1/29.full.

42. Palma-Carlos, A. M. Branco-Ferreira, and M. Palma-Carlos. "Allergic rhinitis and asthma: more similarities than differences." *Allerg Immunol (Paris)*. 33, no. 6 (2001): 237–41.
   http://www.ncbi.nlm.nih.gov/pubmed/11505808

43. Panicker, Radhakrishna,. Nermina Arifhodzic, Mona Al Ahmad, and Seham Ahmed Ali. "Association and symptom characteristics of irritable bowel syndrome among bronchial asthma patients in Kuwait." *Ann Thorac Med*. 5, no. 1 (2010):37–42.
   https://www.ncbi.nlm.nih.gov/pmc/articles/PMC2841807/

44. Powell, Nick, , Benedict Huntley, Thomas Beech, William Knight, Hannah Knight, and Christopher J Corrigan . "Increased prevalence of gastrointestinal symptoms in patients with allergic disease." *Postgrad Med J*. 83 (2007): 182–186.
   https://www.ncbi.nlm.nih.gov/pmc/articles/PMC2599996/pdf/182.pdf

45. European Academy of Allergy & Clinical Immunology. "What is food hypersensitivity?" 2014.
   http://www.eaaci.org/400-resources/what-is-food-allergy/1873-what-is-food-hypersensitivity.html

46. Wang, Julie & Andrew Liu. "Food allergies and asthma." *Curr Opin Allergy Clin Immunol*. 11, no. 3 (2011): 249–254.
   https://www.ncbi.nlm.nih.gov/pmc/articles/PMC3155248/

47. Wark, P, S.L. Johnston, J.L. Simpson, M.J. Hensley, and P.G. Gibson. "Chlamydia pneumoniae immunoglobulin A reactivation and airway inflammation in acute asthma." *European Respiratory Journal*. 20 (2002):834–84.
   http://erj.ersjournals.com/content/20/4/834

THE MECHANISM OF ALLERGY

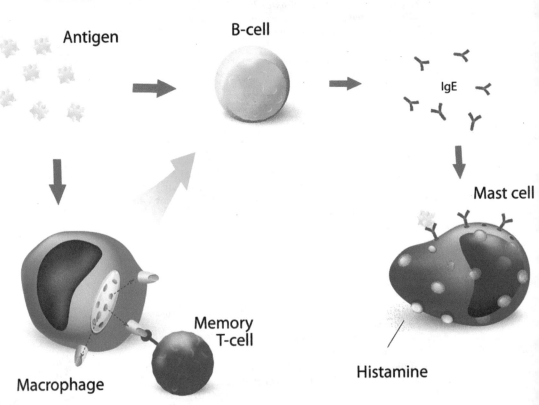

Antigen

B-cell

IgE

Mast cell

Macrophage

Memory
T-cell

Histamine

PART TWO

The immune system as it relates to asthma and allergies

Although the immune system performs vital functions in the body, the clinical symptoms observed in cases of asthma and allergies are a result of inappropriate reactions of the immune system. In this part, I discuss the basic components and functioning of the immune system, and how the immune system becomes dysfunctional in cases of asthma and allergies.

THE MECHANISM OF ALLERGY

Antigen

B-cell

IgE

Mast cell

Memory T-cell

Macrophage

Histamine

Copyright: Designua

CHAPTER 4
How the immune system works

CHAPTER 5
The inflammatory immune response

CHAPTER 4

MECHANISM OF ALLERGY

How the immune system works

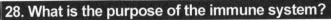
The basic function of the immune system is to protect the body against harmful microorganisms, their products, and toxins. The body has to be able to distinguish "self" which consists of the body's tissues, from "non-self" which are materials foreign to the body.

A basic understanding of the immune system is important in understanding many aspects of asthma and allergies, including diagnosis and treatments.

29. What are the main components of the immune system?

Phagocytes are white blood cells that engulf pathogens and other foreign material. They are an essential part of the innate immune system.

NOTE

The immune system is broadly divided into two branches: cellular and humoral. Cellular immunity is carried out by the white blood cells (lymphocytes), and humoral immunity is carried out by antibodies that circulate in the blood. There are five types of white blood cells that vary in importance in asthma and allergies.

- Antigen presenting cells (APCs) include dendritic cells and macrophages that are found in the epithelial lining of the bronchi. These cells constantly monitor the environment for potential pathogens and other foreign material, collectively known as antigens. When found, the antigens are engulfed, broken down in the cell, and displayed as fragments on the cell surface. For this reason, these cells are known as antigen presenting cells.
- Inflammatory mediators are chemical substances that play a vital role in communicating among immune cells and stimulating their activities. Chemokines are important in the recruitment of inflammatory cells into the airways and are mainly expressed in airway epithelial cells. Cytokines direct and modify the inflammatory response. Leukotrienes are potent bronchoconstrictors derived mainly from mast cells. Nitric oxide is produced in airway epithelial cells; it is

a potent vasodilator (expansion or stretching of blood vessel interiors). A test for exhaled nitric oxide is being developed as a diagnostic tool.

- T-cells or T lymphocytes play a central role in cell-mediated immunity. Of major importance to asthma and allergies are the helper T cells (Th2 cells), so-called because they help other white blood cells in immunologic processes. Helper T-cells have receptor proteins on their surfaces that bind specifically to antigen fragments on APCs. After binding, the Th2 cells are stimulated to initiate the immune response. This initial response involves the activation of B-cells as described in the next section. Typically, the first exposure to allergen does not result in an allergic reaction. This exposure is known as the sensitization phase.

- B-cells are produced in the bone marrow. Once a B-cell is activated by Th2 cells, they differentiate into plasma cells, which produce and secrete antibodies that then enter the blood. Antibodies are very specific to each antigen (allergen). IgE antibodies (see the following discussion) function by binding to specific receptor sites on other cells, notably mast cells, basophils, and eosinophils. When the antigen reenters the body, it binds to the antibody triggering the release of chemical mediators of inflammation.

- Antibodies are proteins known as immunoglobulins and are divided into five classes, three of which are important in the asthmatic process.

  IgE antibodies are recognized to be the principal players in allergies, as most allergy sufferers have an atopic (inherited) tendency to overproduce these antibodies. IgE antibodies bind to receptor sites on mast cells.

  IgG antibodies account for the largest portion of antibodies in the body. IgG has gained the reputation of reducing allergy by competing with and blocking the binding sites for IgE, thereby reducing the activation of IgE. However, there is some evidence for specific IgE receptor sites, indicating that IgG may play a direct role in allergic inflammation and anaphylaxis.

  IgA antibodies are the primary antibodies of the mucus membrane surfaces, including the mucosal surfaces of the respiratory bronchi.

- Mast cells, basophils, and eosinophils have many of the same receptors and release the same cytokines but have different effects in the body. These cells are central to bringing about the effects of allergic inflammation. Mast cells are found in the bronchial epithelium, while basophils are in the circulation in the vicinity of the epithelium. Mast cells are among the first cells an antigen encounters as it enters the lungs. When mast cells are coated with a specific IgE antibody against the antigen, the subsequent binding releases histamine, resulting in symptoms of allergy. Eosinophils are recruited from other parts of the body by chemical messengers released by mast cells, and increase in numbers during the allergic process. Eosinophils have large granules within their cells that normally release toxins to act against parasitic infections but act inappropriately during allergic reactions.

> The allergic response takes place in two steps: an initiation step where an incoming allergen stimulates T helper cells, and a second step with the formation of specific Ig antibodies that cause an allergic reaction during a second encounter with the antigen.
>
> NOTE

30. How does the immune system malfunction in asthma and allergies?

Allergic asthma is an overreaction to environmental substances that are harmless to the body. On a cellular level, the condition results from an inappropriate stimulation of dendritic cells by harmless airborne substances leading to increased production of Th2 cells and IgE antibodies. The exact reasons for this stimulation are still under study.

CHAPTER
MECHANISM OF ALLERGY
5 *The inflammatory immune response*

Memory T-cell

Mast cell

Histamine

31. How does an allergic response work?

The following discussion was obtained from the website of the National Institute of Allergy and Infectious Diseases. This article is an excellent summary of the immune system basis of allergy and asthma conditions.

In allergy-prone people, initial encounters with an allergy-triggering substance, or allergen, prompt changes in the immune system that eventually may lead to allergy symptoms. This stage is called sensitization. When an allergy-prone person inhales pollen, for example, immune cells in the lining of the nose or lungs engulf the pollen allergen and process it into small fragments. These cells, called antigen-presenting cells (APCs), display the allergen fragments on their surfaces.

When white blood cells called type 2 T helper (Th2) cells come into contact with the allergen fragments on APCs, they become activated. The Th2 cells then interact with immune cells known as B cells and release chemical signals that help the B cells develop into antibody-producing plasma cells. These plasma cells make large amounts of a type of antibody called immunoglobulin E (IgE). Each IgE molecule is specific to a particular allergen. IgE produced after exposure to grass pollen, for example, is specific for grass and will not cause a reaction to ragweed pollen. IgE binds to the surface of specialized cells called mast cells that reside in the tissues, particularly in the skin and at mucous membranes.

When a person who has made IgE to an allergen is exposed to the same allergen again, the allergen interacts with IgE on the surface of mast cells. The binding of allergen to IgE triggers these cells to release histamine, leukotrienes, and other chemicals, leading to allergy symptoms. For example, histamine acts on nerves, which can cause sneezing, an itchy feeling, and a runny nose. Leukotrienes contribute to the widening of blood vessels, which can result in swelling inside the nose, causing a stuffy nose. In people with asthma, leukotrienes can make the muscles surrounding the airways contract, narrowing the airways and causing an exacerbation. Drugs known as antihistamines or leukotriene receptor antagonists block the action of histamine and leukotrienes and can provide relief from allergy symptoms.

Reexposure to an allergen also causes mast cells and Th2 cells to release chemical messengers that attract and activate other inflammatory cells, such as eosinophils and basophils, which release more chemicals and cause allergy symptoms to worsen and last longer. Nasal steroids are anti-inflammatory medications that help decrease the inflammatory cell responses to an allergen.

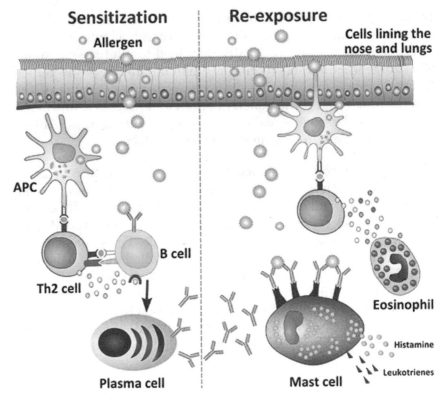

Sensitization

Allergen

Re-exposure

Cells lining the nose and lungs

APC

Th2 cell

B cell

Plasma cell

Mast cell

Eosinophil

Histamine

Leukotrienes

▲ **Figure 5.1**
Summary of allergic sensitization
Credit: National Institute of Allergy and Infectious Diseases

During sensitization, an antigen-presenting cell (APC) picks up the allergen and presents part of it to a Th2 cell, which helps a B cell become a plasma cell. Plasma cells produce allergen-specific antibodies called IgE, which binds to mast cells. When allergen returns, mast cells release histamine and other chemicals. Also, Th2 cells release many different chemicals that attract inflammatory cells such as eosinophils. The inflammatory cells cause allergy symptoms such as sneezing, mucus production, swelling, itching, runny nose, coughing, and wheezing.

32. What is the central role of IgE in asthma?

Allergy and asthma patients are noted for having an increased production of IgE while normal people do not.

Immune deficiency is a situation where the person's immune system is incompletely developed or even absent, so the immune response to pathogens or other foreign substances is inadequate. Development of the immune response in childhood is an active process begun during the fetal period and continuing during the first years of the child's life. The observed

For a video on the development of new therapies based on an understanding of increased production of IgE in allergies, visit: https://www.nationaljewish.org/healthinfo/conditions/asthma/causes

symptoms of allergy are a result of a combination of the person's genetic predisposition to asthma, as well as the exposure to activating allergens and microbial antigens.

Immune-deficient people can be divided into two groups, primary and secondary. Primary immune deficiency is genetic in origin and relates to how the immune system develops. Secondary immune deficiency is caused by environmental factors not directly related to the immune system. Examples include chemotherapy, radiation, severe burns, malnutrition, and kidney disease. Once considered rare diseases involving severely ill individuals, primary immunodeficiencies now appear to be more common than previously thought. In fact, it is estimated that 1 of 500 people have the most common immunodeficiency—selective IgA immunodeficiency.

The Diagnosis section will describe when immunodeficiency should be considered, as well as the warning signs that may indicate immunodeficiency.

34. What is the working definition of asthma put forth by the National Heart, Lung, and Blood Institute?

With a basic understanding of the immune system as it relates to asthma, a more comprehensive definition of asthma can be stated as follows:

"Asthma is a chronic inflammatory disorder of the airways in which many cells and cellular elements play a role: in particular, mast cells, eosinophils, T lymphocytes, macrophages, neutrophils, and epithelial cells. In susceptible individuals, this inflammation

The National Heart, Lung, and Blood Institute, through their National Asthma Education and Prevention Program prepared an excellent report in 2007 entitled: "Expert Panel Report 3: Guidelines for the Diagnosis and Management of Asthma." This book refers heavily from this report, and will be referred to as "EPR-3." Please go to: https://www.nhlbi.nih.gov/files/docs/guidelines/asthgdln.pdf

ON THE WEB

causes recurrent episodes of wheezing, breathlessness, chest tightness, and coughing, particularly at night or in the early morning. These episodes are usually associated with widespread but variable airflow obstruction that is often reversible either spontaneously or with treatment. The inflammation also causes an associated increase in the existing bronchial hyperresponsiveness to a variety of stimuli. Reversibility of airflow limitation may be incomplete in some patients with asthma."

References

REFERENCES
MECHANISM OF ALLERGY

CHAPTER 4

1. American Academy of Allergy, Asthma & Immunology. "Asthma 1. Hoffmann, Franzika, Ender F, Schmudde I, Lewkowich I, Köhl J, König P, and Laumonnier Y. "Origin, localization, and immunoregulatory properties of pulmonary phagocytes in allergic asthma." *Frontiers in Immunology.* 7, no. 107 (2016):1–16.
https://www.ncbi.nlm.nih.gov/pubmed/?term=Origin%2C+Localization%2C+and+Immunoregulatory+Properties+of+Pulmonary+Phagocytes+in+Allergic+Asthma

CHAPTER 5

2. National Institute of Allergy and Infectious Diseases. "Allergic diseases." National Institute of Health. (2016).
https://www.niaid.nih.gov/topics/allergicdiseases/Pages/default.aspx

3. Szczawinska-Poplonyk, Aleksandra. "An overlapping syndrome of allergy and immune deficiency in children." *J Allergy.* 2012 (2012) Article ID 658279.
https://www.hindawi.com/journals/ja/2012/658279/

3. National Asthma Education and Prevention Program. "Expert Panel Report 3: Guidelines for the Diagnosis and Management of Asthma." National Heart, Lung, and Blood Institute. (2007).
http://www.nhlbi.nih.gov/files/docs/guidelines/asthgdln.pdf

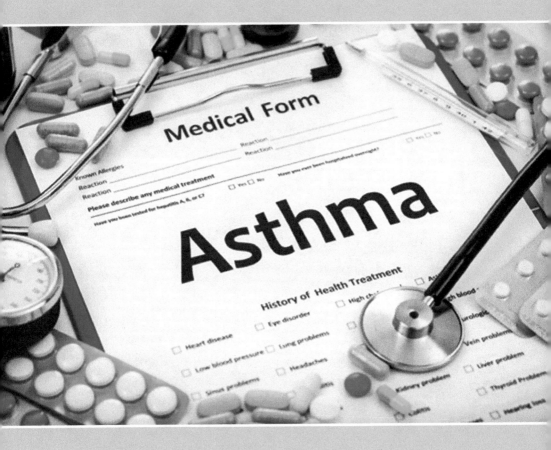

PART THREE

Diagnosis of Asthma

Part Three will discuss the methods used to diagnosis asthma including consultation with the patient and the various diagnostic tests.

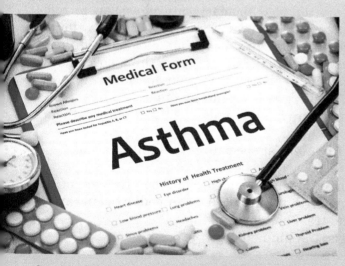

CHAPTER 6
Seeing your doctor

CHAPTER 7
Diagnostic tests for asthma

Copyright: Shutterstock

Seeing your doctor

35. Who is a primary care physician?

The first physician you see will most likely be a primary care physician and could be a family practitioner, an internist, or a pediatrician. All primary care physicians have completed four years of medical school followed by three years of residency training. The kind of specialty that the primary care physician enters is determined by differences in the residency training he or she receives. Family practice physicians focus on the entire spectrum of medical issues that might be encountered by the members of a family unit. Family practice grew out of what was known as general practice. Internal medicine physicians (also known as internists) focus solely on diseases facing adults. Pediatricians are primary care physicians for children during the four primary stages of development from infancy (birth – 1 year), early childhood (1–4 years), middle childhood (4–10 years), and adolescence (11–18 years).

Your physician makes an asthma diagnosis based on four means: a physical exam, a detailed medical history, your overall health, and diagnostic tests.

NOTE

36. Who is an asthma specialist?

It may be necessary for your primary care physician to refer you to an asthma specialist. An asthma specialist has similar training as a primary care physician but has an additional 2–3 years of more specialized training. An asthma specialist is known by different names according to their specialty:

- Allergist – An allergist is a pediatrician or internist who specializes in allergy and immunology, including asthma and allergic asthma.
- Internist – An internist specializes in adult internal medicine.
- Pediatrician – A pediatrician specializes in the care of children from birth through college. A pediatrician can diagnose and treat childhood asthma.
- Pulmonologist – A pulmonologist specializes in respiratory diseases.

37. When would you be referred to an asthma specialist?

The National Heart, Lung, and Blood Institute has prepared guidelines for referral of a patient to an asthma specialist.

- Patient is not meeting the goals of asthma therapy after 3–6 months of treatment.
- Patient has had a life-threatening asthma exacerbation.
- Patient's response to treatment is limited, incomplete, or very slow, and poor control interferes with the patient's quality of life.
- Coexisting illnesses and/or their treatment complicate the management of asthma.
- Other conditions are complicating asthma or its diagnosis.
- Patient experiences signs and symptoms that are not typical.
- Patient has recurrent absences from school or work due to asthma.
- Oral corticosteroids (an asthma medication) are frequently required.
- Patient requires additional education and guidance on complications of therapy, problems with adherence to medications, or allergen avoidance.
- Patient requires multiple medications on a long-term basis.
- Patient requires confirmation that an occupational or environmental substance is provoking or contributing to asthma.
- Patients have significant psychological or family problems that interfere with their asthma therapy.
- Patient is being considered for immunotherapy (allergy shots).

38. How should you prepare for a visit to your physician?

During your first visit to the doctor's office, you will probably be required to fill out a questionnaire. Your physician may even provide you with a questionnaire in advance. Be prepared to provide the following details:

- Provide your insurance plan, and make sure the physician participates in the plan.
- Discuss medical problems you have or had, and their duration.

- List medications you are taking, and their dosages.
- Indicate if you have relatives with asthma, allergies, sinusitis, rhinitis, eczema, and nasal polyps.
- Describe symptoms you are experiencing (see Questions 39 & 40).
- Discuss if you often exposed to airborne irritants such as tobacco smoke, chemical fumes, or dust.
- Indicate if you have pets in the home.

39. What are the common signs and symptoms of asthma?

- Wheezing – high-pitched whistling sounds when breathing out – especially in children. (Lack of wheezing and a normal chest examination do not exclude asthma.)
- History of any of the following:
  o Cough, worse particularly at night
  o Recurrent wheeze
  o Recurrent difficulty in breathing
  o Recurrent chest tightness
- Symptoms occur or worsen in the presence of:
  o Exercise (appears out of alignment)
  o Viral infection
  o Animals with fur or hair
  o House-dust mites (in mattresses, pillows, upholstered furniture, carpets)
  o Mold
  o Smoke (tobacco, wood)
  o Pollen
  o Changes in weather
  o Strong emotional expression (laughing or crying hard)
  o Airborne chemicals or dusts
  o Menstrual cycles
- Symptoms occur or worsen at night, awakening the patient

Other nonspecific symptoms in infants or young children may be a history of recurrent bronchitis, bronchiolitis, or pneumonia; a persistent cough with colds; and/or recurrent croup or chest rattling.

40. What are some unusual asthma symptoms?

- Rapid breathing
- Sighing
- Fatigue

- Difficulty sleeping
- Anxiety

41. How does the doctor look for signs of asthma during a physical exam?

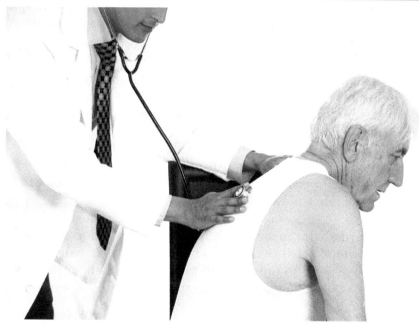

▲ **Figure 6.1**
Physician examining patient for asthma
Shutterstock Standard License
Copyright: pathdoc

As we have been discussing, asthma is a complex disease that can be associated with many other conditions. The doctor's physical exam, therefore, can be quite comprehensive. A typical exam may include:

- Ear exam. The doctor will examine your ears to look for signs of infection or fluid.
- Eye exam. The doctor will look for redness, swelling, inflammation, or discharge. These symptoms may indicate allergic rhinitis.
- Nose exam. The doctor will examine both the inside and outside of your nose. Your doctor will look for swelling of normal structures on the inside of the nose. He or she will also check the color and consistency of the nasal lining and the nature of any nasal discharge. Finally,

he or she will look for signs of bleeding; and look for any abnormal structures present, such as a nasal polyp or a foreign body. The exam of the outside of your nose looks for a horizontal crease across the lower one-third of the nose (called an "allergic crease") that forms as a result of rubbing the nose to relieve nasal itching and congestion. Also, your doctor will watch for itching of the nose.

- Mouth exam. Your doctor will look in your mouth to assess the health and hygiene of your gums and teeth; look for postnasal drip (amount, color, consistency); and check for redness or inflammation of your throat, and the size and quality of your tonsils.

- Lung exam. He will listen to your lungs (front and back of the chest) for wheezes, crackles, congestion, or any other abnormal sounds. Also, he will likely have you do different breathing maneuvers (deep breaths, blow out breath, etc.) while he listens.

- Chest. Your doctor will take a look at your chest for abnormalities in size or shape. He or she will ask you to breathe to see if the chest is moving symmetrically (both sides moving in unison) and to see if it is using accessory (extra) muscles to breathe. Your doctor will be listening for any signs of wheezing during breathing.

- Neck. The physician examines your neck for rashes, tightness, and signs of itching. The physician will also feel your neck for signs of abnormally swollen lymph nodes or enlarged thyroid.

- Heart. Your doctor will listen to your heart for abnormal sounds (murmurs) or rhythm. Asthma medications can cause heart palpitations.

- Abdomen. The doctor will feel your abdomen for pain or tenderness, signs of an enlarged liver or spleen, or any other abnormal masses. A distended stomach can be a sign of asthma. He will also listen for normal bowel sounds.

- Skin. The skin exam looks for any signs of allergy, such as rashes, eczema, or hives. Some facial features may indicate allergic disease: Allergic shiners are dark circles under the eyes due to swelling and discoloration from the congestion of small vessels beneath the skin in this area. This condition is due to allergic rhinitis. Dennie-Morgan lines are crease-like wrinkles that form under the lower eyelid folds. This condition can occur in young children with nasal allergies or atopic dermatitis. Nasal allergies may promote swelling of the adenoids resulting in a droopy appearance to the face.

- Postnasal drip. Children may experience a constant postnasal drip and repeated sore throats from allergic mucus building up and being discharged into the throat. Serious nasal allergies also reduce the sense of taste and smell.

42. How is a diagnosis of asthma established?

The following broad outline for diagnosis is presented in "NHLBI Guidelines for the Diagnosis and Management of Asthma."

To establish a diagnosis of asthma, the clinician should determine that:
- Episodic symptoms of airflow obstruction or airway hyperresponsiveness are present.
- Airflow obstruction is at least partially reversible.
- Alternative diagnoses are excluded.

Recommended methods to establish the diagnosis are
- Detailed medical history.
- Physical exam focusing on the upper respiratory tract, chest, and skin.
- Spirometry to demonstrate obstruction in the lungs, and to assess reversibility. The spirometry test can be performed in adults, and in children 5 years of age or older. Reversibility is determined either by an increase in FEV1 of ≥12% from baseline or by an increase ≥10% of predicted FEV1 after inhalation of a short-acting bronchodilator (The spirometry test is described in Question 49).
- Additional tests as necessary to exclude alternate diagnoses.

43. What are key indicators a physician considers in making a diagnosis?

The following indicators are not diagnostic by themselves, but the presence of multiple key indicators increases the probability of a diagnosis of asthma.

Diagnosis of asthma is dependent on specific symptoms, physical exam findings, and specialized lung functions results.

The task of your physician is to determine if the symptoms you are experiencing are due to asthma or some other condition. Based on the physician's medical training and previous experience, he or she will come up with a list of possible diagnoses. When the patient's medical history or physical examination does not lead to a definite conclusion, the physician will order tests that could further differentiate among possible conditions. Spirometry is an important tool to establish a diagnosis of asthma. The physician may even make a provisional diagnosis and prescribe an asthma treatment to see if the medication alleviates the symptoms.

44. What is differential diagnosis as it relates to asthma?

Differential diagnosis refers to examination for comorbid conditions (occur together with asthma) or for conditions that are similar to asthma.

- Cardiac asthma is a misnomer since it is not asthma. The condition is due to congestive heart failure which causes fluid to collect in the lungs around and within the bronchial tubes. The symptoms could include a sudden onset of difficult breathing, coughing, and wheezing that resemble asthma. The symptoms occur almost exclusively late at night or early morning when the patient is lying down. A large portion of elderly patients with congestive heart failure have symptoms of cardiac asthma.

A differential diagnosis is a systematic diagnostic method used to identify the presence of a particular disease where multiple alternatives are possible.

- Vocal cord dysfunction (VCD) – This condition is also known as laryngeal asthma and is due to an abnormal closure of the vocal cords when the patient breathes in. As air is drawn through the constricted opening of the vocal cords a wheezing sound resembling asthma is produced. In asthma, breathing is difficult due to constriction of the bronchial tubes, while in VCD the vocal cords tighten making breathing difficult. Furthermore, VCD causes more difficulty breathing in than breathing out, while in asthma the reverse is true.
- Nonasthmatic eosinophilic bronchitis (NAEB) is a rare disease characterized by airway inflammation due to eosinophils, similar to that seen in asthma. However, in

contrast to asthma, nonasthmatic eosinophilic bronchitis is not associated with variable airflow limitation or airway hyperresponsiveness. This condition is a common cause of chronic cough. Patients with NAEB do not respond to corticosteroid therapy (a common asthma medication).

- Foreign body aspiration is a particular concern for young children. The aspirated object can lodge in the larynx or trachea and can be life-threatening if it is large enough. The most common symptom is wheezing. It may be necessary to remove the object by bronchoscopy. The offending object is often food, but a wide variety of objects have been found.

- A variety of benign or malignant tumors can cause symptoms of asthma if they block the airways.

- Pulmonary embolism is a blood clot that originates in the venous system of the lower extremities and travels to the bifurcation of the pulmonary artery where it lodges and constricts the bronchi. This condition can cause many symptoms including wheezing and cough.

- Chronic obstructive pulmonary disease (COPD) – This disease was discussed in Question 20. COPD can result in both bronchitis and emphysema (lung diseases). Airflow obstruction in COPD is not completely reversible. Patients with COPD can have signs and symptoms similar to asthma including cough, breathlessness, and wheezing. Physical examination is more specific and sensitive for advanced COPD, compared to mild or moderate COPD. Diagnosis of COPD is made with spirometry. The data obtained with this test allows for the calculation of the FEV_1/FVC ratio (forced expiratory volume in 1 second divided by forced vital capacity). COPD is diagnosed when the FEV_1/FVC ratio is less than 70% of control (the spirometry test will be discussed in Question 49).

- Gastroesophageal reflux disease (GERD) – This disease was discussed in Question 21. When symptoms and medical history suggest GERD, it is important to prevent or minimize the reflux of stomach acid and bile into the esophagus that could be aspirated into the bronchi. The physician could make a tentative diagnosis of GERD and prescribe a specialized GERD medication such as a proton pump inhibitor or H2 blocker to reduce the generation of stomach acid. When the diagnosis is uncertain or more complicated, the physician could order tests to evaluate the condition of the esophagus. These tests could include a barium study, upper endoscopy, pH study, or manometry.

Allergic rhinitis and sinusitis are upper airway infections that are often associated with asthma.

45. How is cough related to asthma?

Cough in asthma can be classified into three categories: cough-variant asthma, cough-predominant asthma, and cough that persists despite standard therapy. These conditions are examples of chronic cough, defined as cough lasting for 8 weeks or longer. Chronic cough can also be due to rhinitis. Cough variant asthma (CVA) is a subclass of asthma in which the dominant and usually only symptom is a dry, non-productive cough. A non-productive

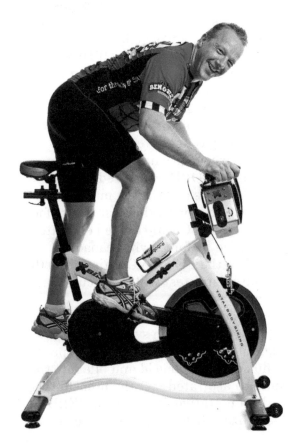

◀ **Figure 6.2**
Indoor bike
Credit: WyrdLight.com/
Wikimedia
Creative Commons License:
CC BY-SA 3.0

cough does not expel any mucus from the respiratory tract. A cough may be provoked by cold air or viral infections of the upper respiratory tract. In cough-predominant asthma, cough is the most predominant symptom but other symptoms are also present such as breathlessness or wheeze. Airway hyperresponsiveness tends to be milder in CVA than in "classical" or more typical asthma, but CVA patients may be more difficult to manage. CVA is one of the most common causes of chronic cough. About 30–40 % of adult patients with CVA, if not adequately treated, may progress to the more typical asthma.

Cough is the most predominant symptom in cough-predominant asthma, but other symptoms are also present such as breathlessness and/or wheezing.

Conditions other than asthma can cause chronic cough including GERD, postnasal drip, and cough following a viral respiratory disease.

46. What is exercise-induced asthma?

The preferred term for this condition is exercise-induced bronchoconstriction (EIB) since exercise does not cause asthma. Exercise-induced bronchoconstriction (EIB) can be defined as temporary, reversible bronchoconstriction that happens during and after strenuous exercise. More than 10% of the general population and up to 90% of people previously diagnosed with asthma have EIB.

The symptoms of EIB may begin during exercise and will usually be worse 5 to 10 minutes after stopping exercise. Symptoms most often resolve in another 20 to 30 minutes and can range from mild to severe. Symptoms include a dry, nagging cough, wheezing, shortness of breath, and chest tightness. EIB can be a particularly serious problem in athletes involved in competitive sports, as prolonged periods of strenuous activity can magnify the problem.

EIB symptoms are often triggered by exercises that involve breathing cold, dry air. When a person finishes exercising, the airway responds by dilating blood vessels to warm the airways. The resulting engorgement of the airways causes the symptoms of asthma, including bronchoconstriction and the release of inflammatory mediators.

Diagnosis of EIB can be difficult if the symptoms only appear during or immediately following exercise. The diagnostic test for asthma, spirometry, will appear normal for people in the resting state even if they have EIB. For competitive athletes, further diagnostic tests could be necessary.

The prevention and treatment will be discussed in detail in Part Four. These topics are particularly important for athletes.

47. What is Samter's Triad?

Aspirin Exacerbated Respiratory Disease (AERD) is also known as Samter's Triad) – The term comes from a triad of symptoms associated with asthma: bronchospasm, nasal polyps, and increased sensitivity to aspirin or other non-steroidal anti-inflammatory drugs (NSAIDs).

NSAIDs are commonly used to treat pain, fever, and inflammation. NSAIDs act by inhibiting the activity of cyclooxygenase 1 enzyme (COX-1). They are available over-the-counter and by prescription. Common NSAIDs include acetylsalicylic acid (aspirin), ibuprofen (Advil, Motrin), and naproxen (Aleve). They are also commonly included in cough and cold medications.

AERD sufferers can have nasal conditions in addition to polyps, including rhinitis (inflammation of the nose), sneezing, nasal drip, and congestion. AERD is a chronic condition that can follow a protracted course even after NSAIDs are avoided. Patients typically develop AERD symptoms in early adulthood. Approximately 10% of people with asthma have AERD.

The symptoms of respiratory reactions in this syndrome are hypersensitivity reactions to NSAIDs rather than the typically described true allergic reactions that trigger other common allergen-induced asthma, rhinitis, or hives. The NSAID-induced reactions do not appear to involve the common mediators of true allergic reactions. NSAIDs are thought to exert their effect on inducing asthma through increased production of pro-inflammatory chemical mediators known as leukotrienes.

Nasal polyps are common noncancerous growths that form in the nose or sinuses. They are usually found around the area where the sinuses open into the nasal cavity. Nasal polyps may cause no symptoms unless they grow so large that they block normal drainage from the sinuses.

Treatments and surgeries for AERD, including aspirin desensitization, will be discussed in the Treatments section.

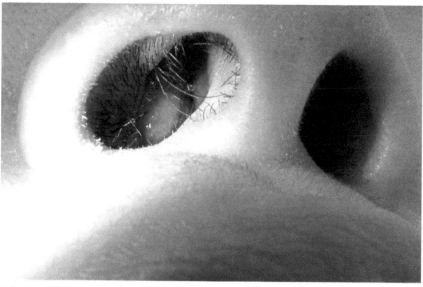

▲ **Figure 6.3**
Nasal polyps
Credit: Mathieu MD
Creative Commons License: CC BY-SA 3.0

Diagnostic Tests for Asthma

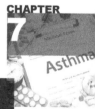

48. Why would a physician order diagnostic tests for asthma?

Diagnostic tests provide an objective means of establishing a diagnosis of asthma by characterizing the degree of lung impairment and by excluding other diagnoses.

49. What are pulmonary function tests?

Pulmonary function tests are considered to be the most reliable means of evaluating the extent to which your lung function is limited or affected. Pulmonary function tests are used both in the diagnosis of asthma and for monitoring the control of asthma. Pulmonary function tests help to determine whether there is airflow obstruction, its severity, and whether it is reversible over the short term (can improve with treatment).

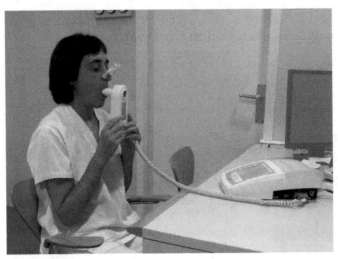

Spirometry (meaning the measuring of breath) is used to detect and measure the degree of airflow obstruction. The test is conducted using a device known as a spirometer. Two important measurements are obtained in spirometry, forced expiratory volume and forced vital capacity.

Forced expiratory volume (FEV) is considered to be the most important measurement in the diagnosis and management of asthma. In the FEV test, the patient takes in the deepest breath they can, and then exhales into the sensor as hard as possible, for as long as possible. The results are displayed on a graph relating volume (in liters) expired versus time in seconds.

FEV_1 is the volume of air expired in 1 second. Average values for FEV_1 in healthy people depend mainly on sex and age. Values of between 80% and 120% of the average value are considered normal. Predicted normal values for FEV1 can be calculated online and depend on age, sex, height, mass, and ethnicity. The maneuver is highly dependent on patient cooperation and effort and is normally repeated at least three times to ensure reproducibility. Due to the patient cooperation required, spirometry can only be used on children old enough to comprehend and follow the instructions given (6 years old or more), and only on patients who can understand and follow instructions.

Your doctor may order a bronchodilator to be given as part of spirometry. A bronchodilator is an inhaled medication that may dilate, or open up, your airways. Spirometry is often done before and after the bronchodilator to show any response to the medicine. Your response may help your doctor find out what kind and how much, if any, airway disease you may have, and whether you need medication to improve your breathing.

Forced Vital Capacity (FVC) measures the total volume of air exhaled after taking in as deep a breath as possible. FEV, on the other hand, measures the volume of air exhaled after a specific period, usually 1 second. This measurement is used to calculate the ratio of FEV_1 to FVC (FEV_1/FVC). A reduced ratio indicates an obstruction to the flow of air from the lungs. In healthy adults, this should be approximately 70–85% (declining with age). Since asthma reduces the openings of bronchial tubes, the time required for the complete expiration of air from the lungs is increased from a normal of 5–6 seconds to as long as 14 seconds. FEV_1 is diminished to a greater extent than FVC in asthmatics resulting in a reduced value (less than 80%, often to around 45%).

Due to the difficulty of some patients (older persons in particular) to totally exhaust the air in their lungs, the National Institutes of Health has proposed the adoption of FEV_6 (forced expiratory volume in 6 seconds) as a substitute for FVC. FEV_6 has been shown to be equivalent to FVC for identifying obstructive and restrictive lung function. FEV_6 is more reproducible and less physically demanding than FVC.

Sometimes, to assess the reversibility of a particular condition, a bronchodilator is administered to counteract the effects of the bronchoconstrictor before repeating the spirometry tests. This procedure is commonly referred to as a reversibility test, or a post-bronchodilator test (post-BD), and may help in distinguishing asthma from chronic obstructive pulmonary disease. COPD patients may show less improvement in FEV_1 after taking a bronchodilator.

Flow volume loops. This test is a modification of the basic spirometry test that adds rapid and maximal inhalation breathing maneuvers. This test can detect obstruction in the upper airway that can be due to vocal cord paralysis or dysfunction or if there are questions about coexisting COPD.

Peak flow meters are inexpensive, portable, handheld devices for those with asthma that are used to measure how well air moves out of your lungs. Peak flow meters work by measuring how fast air moves out of the lungs when you exhale forcefully after inhaling fully. This air flow rate is known as peak expiratory flow. Peak flow measures the flow of air through the larger conducting airways in asthma. Peak expiratory flow is measured as volume of air expired per minute.

Peak flow meters are not as accurate as spirometry but are more convenient. As such, they have found more application for monitoring asthma rather than for diagnosis. Peak flow meters are more useful for patients with moderate to severe asthma, or for young children who cannot take the spirometry test. They can be used for measurements in the home environment to aid in gauging responses to treatments, improve asthma control, and to reduce exacerbations.

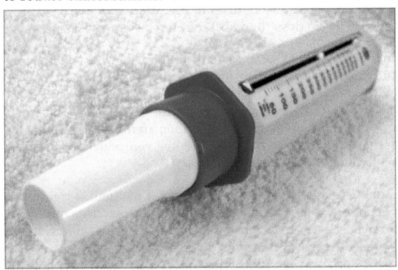

▲ **Figure 7.2**
Example of a peak flow meter
Source: https://commons.wikimedia.org/wiki/File:Peak_flow_meter_horiz.jpg
Author: Tomhannen; released into the Public Domain

A bronchoprovocation challenge test may be considered when asthma is suspected, but spirometry is normal or near normal. Bronchoprovocation can be conducted with the chemicals methacholine or histamine, or even cold air or vigorous exercise. Bronchoprovocation provokes bronchoconstriction or narrowing of the airways. The test is valuable for excluding asthma. If the test is negative, asthma is ruled out. If the test is positive, there is a good likelihood that the patient has asthma. However, not all people that test positive for the test have asthma.

A positive methacholine bronchoprovocation test is diagnostic for the presence of airway hyperresponsiveness, a characteristic feature of asthma that also can be present in other conditions (e.g., allergic rhinitis, cystic fibrosis, and COPD, among others). Thus, although a positive test is consistent with asthma, a negative bronchoprovocation may be more helpful to rule out asthma.

50. When would a chest X-ray be considered?

A chest X-ray is usually done to rule out other conditions that may be causing your symptoms, as people with asthma will usually have a normal chest X-ray. Emphysema causes holes in lung tissue, while tumors could indicate lung cancer.

51. What is a nitric oxide test?

Nitric oxide, a gaseous molecule, performs many functions in the lungs and airways, including dilating blood vessels and bronchi, transmitting nerve impulses and reducing inflammation. In asthmatics, increased nitric oxide in the exhaled breath indicates inflammation due to eosinophils. The nitric oxide test involves a person exhaling into a machine that measures the amount of nitric oxide. The fractional nitric oxide concentration (FENO) is then calculated. A high level of FENO might be useful to rule in a diagnosis of asthma, but a lower level might not be useful to rule asthma out.

The nitric oxide test is also useful as a follow-up and as a guide to therapy in adults and children with asthma. People with high FENO levels are more likely to respond positively to corticosteroid treatments for asthma. The test is also useful in monitoring the progress of asthma treatments.

52. What is a sputum eosinophils test?

This test looks for eosinophils in the mixture of saliva and mucus (sputum) you discharge during coughing. The test is considered to be a direct measurement of airway inflammation that involves eosinophils (commonly occurring in asthma). The test has been promoted as being a noninvasive, safe, and reproducible method. The test has important therapeutic implications, as patients with inflammation not due to eosinophils respond poorly to treatment with inhaled corticosteroids. The test can also be useful in monitoring the progress of asthma treatments. It is very common for asthma patients also to have sinusitis. Studies have shown that patients with high levels of sputum eosinophils also have greater mucosal thickening of the sinus lining indicating a similar inflammatory process in the two conditions.

Studies have shown a close relationship between the results of the sputum eosinophils test and forced expiratory volume (FEV_1).

53. How do you diagnose allergies?

As we have been discussing, there is a close relationship between asthma and allergies. When your medical history and symptoms indicate the possibility of allergies, your primary physician may refer you to an allergy specialist, known as an allergist or immunologist.

After the allergist reviews your medical history and performs a physical exam, he or she may decide that skin testing is appropriate as a diagnostic aid and does not put you at risk for an asthmatic attack or anaphylaxis. A trained nurse performs the skin testing, and the allergist reads and evaluates the results.

There are two types of skin tests:
- Prick/puncture test: also known as a scratch test. The doctor or nurse will clean the skin on your forearm or back with alcohol. They will then mark and label areas on the skin with a pen. A drop of potential allergen will then be placed on each of the spots. Finally, they will lightly scratch the outer layer of the skin to let in the allergen.
- Intradermal test: This test will only be performed if the scratch test fails to produce a significant positive result.

Using a very thin needle, the doctor or nurse injects a diluted antigen just below the skin surface in a series of rows on the arm. Since the intradermal test involves injecting allergen below the protective surface of the skin, there is a small risk of a widespread systemic reaction.

After either type of test, the area of the skin is observed for about 15 minutes to see if a reaction develops. The "wheal"—a swollen, red, itchy bump and surrounding "flare"—indicates the presence of specific IgE antibody to the allergen tested. A positive test, however, does not prove that the patient is clinically reactive to the allergen. The size of the reaction may correlate with the likelihood that the patient is clinically reactive to the antigen. The reaction usually disappears within 1 hour. Delayed reactions, known as late-phase skin reactions, can develop 3–10 hours after the test, and continue for up to 12 hours after that period. These delayed reactions appear as swollen, red, or numb bumps at the skin test site.

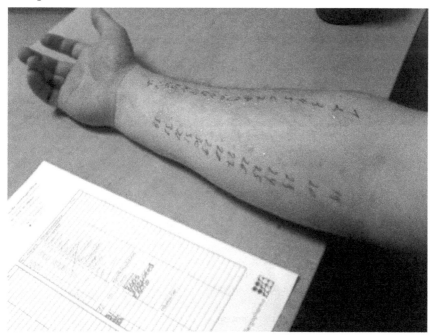

▲ Figure 7.3
Allergy scratch testing
Source: https://commons.wikimedia.org/wiki/File:Allergy_skin_testing.JPG
Author: Wolfgang Ihloff
Creative Commons Attribution Share Alike 3.0 Unported

Blood testing may be necessary for diagnosing asthma when skin testing is not suitable for some patients. The most common blood test used is the enzyme-linked immunosorbent assay or ELISA. Allergy blood testing may be necessary if you:

- Cannot stop taking medications such as antihistamines, steroids, and certain antidepressants that could interfere with test results.
- Have a severe skin condition such as eczema, dermatitis, or psoriasis.
- Have a history of life-threatening allergic reaction (anaphylaxis).
- Have problematic behavioral, physical, or mental problems that prevent cooperating in the skin testing process.

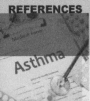

References

CHAPTER 6

1. Asthma and Allergy Foundation of America. "Exercise-induced bronchoconstriction (Asthma)(2015).
   http://www.aafa.org/page/exercise-induced-asthma.aspx

2. *Australian Asthma Handbook.* "Diagnosis of asthma." National Asthma Council Australia. (2017).
   http://www.asthmahandbook.org.au/diagnosis

3. Brightling, C. "Chronic cough due to nonasthmatic eosinophilic bronchitis: ACCP evidence-based clinical practice guidelines." *Chest.* 129, no. 1 (Suppl)(2006):116S–121S.
   https://www.ncbi.nlm.nih.gov/pubmed/?term=Chest.+129%2C+no.+1+(Suppl)(2006)%3A116S-121S

4. Krafczyk, Michael and Chad Asplund. "Exercise-induced bronchoconstriction: diagnosis and management." *American Family Physician.* 84, no. 4(2011):427–434.
   https://www.researchgate.net/profile/Chad_Asplund/publication/51572542_Exercise-Induced_Bronchoconstriction_Diagnosis_and_Management/links/02e7e53c58eb3cab40000000.pdf

5. Lombardo, Thomas and Tinsley Harrison. "Cardiac asthma." *Circulation.* 4 (1951):920-929.
   http://circ.ahajournals.org/content/4/6/920.long

6. Morris, Michael. "Asthma clinical presentation." *Medscape.* Jun. 16, 2016.
   http://emedicine.medscape.com/article/296301-overview

7. Nilmi, Akio. "Cough and asthma." *Curr Respir Med Rev.* 7, no.1(2011):47–54.
   https://www.ncbi.nlm.nih.gov/pmc/articles/PMC3182093/

8. Szezeklik, A. "Mechanism of aspirin-induced asthma." *Allergy.* 52 (1997): 613-619.
   http://onlinelibrary.wiley.com/doi/10.1111/j.1398-9995.1997.tb01039.x/pdf

9. Tidy, Richard. "Diagnosing childhood asthma in primary care." *Patient Platform Limited.* Nov. 29, 2016.
http://patient.info/pdf/1103.pdf#

10. Zeitz, H. "Bronchial asthma, nasal polyps, and aspirin sensitivity: Samter's syndrome." *Clin Chest Med.* 9, no. 4 (1988): 567–76.
https://www.ncbi.nlm.nih.gov/pubmed/3069289

CHAPTER 7

11. Barnes, Peter. "New drugs for asthma." *Semin Respir Crit Care Med.* 33, no. 6 (2012):685–694.
http://www.medscape.com/viewarticle/774255_1
(Requires signing up for a free Medscape account for access).

12. Catley, Matthew. "Dissociated steroids." *The Scientific World Journal.* 7 (2007):421–430.
https://www.hindawi.com/journals/tswj/2007/462054/abs/

13. Coulson, F. and Fryer, A. "Muscarinic acetylcholine receptors and airway diseases." *Pharmacol Ther.* 98, No. 1 (2003):59–69.
https://www.ncbi.nlm.nih.gov/pubmed/12667888

14. Dimov, Vasselin and Thomas Casale. "Immunomodulators for asthma." *Allergy Asthma Immunol Res.* 2, no. 4 (2010):228–234.
https://www.ncbi.nlm.nih.gov/pmc/articles/PMC2946700/pdf/aair-2-228.pdf

15. National Asthma Education and Prevention Program. "Expert Panel Report 3: Guidelines for the Diagnosis and Management of Asthma." National Heart, Lung, and Blood Institute. (2007).
http://www.nhlbi.nih.gov/files/docs/guidelines/asthgdln.pdf

16. Novelli, Federica, Laura Malagrinò, Federico L Dente, and Pierluigi Paggiaro . "Efficacy of anticholinergic drugs in asthma." *Expert Rev Resp Med.* 6, no. 3 (2012):309–319.
http://www.medscape.com/viewarticle/768208

17. Rosenal, Thomas. "Uses and abuses of theophylline." *Canadian Family Physician.* 33 (1987):2575–2579.
https://www.ncbi.nlm.nih.gov/pmc/articles/PMC2218668/pdf/canfamphys00189-0145.pdf

18. Salpeter, Shelley. "Cardioselective beta blocker use in patients with asthma and chronic obstructive pulmonary disease: an evidence-based approach to standards of care." *Cardiovascular Reviews & Reports* 24, no. 11 (2003).
http://www.medscape.com/viewarticle/464040

19. Taylor, D., M, Pijnenburg, A. Smith, and J. Jongste. "Exhaled nitric oxide measurements: clinical application and interpretation." *Thorax.* 61, no. 9 (2006):817–827.
http://thorax.bmj.com/content/61/9/817

20. Walters, J., Wood-Baker, R., and Walters, E. "Long-acting beta2-agonists in asthma: an overview of Cochrane systematic reviews." *Respiratory Medicine.* 99 (2005):384–395.
https://www.ncbi.nlm.nih.gov/pubmed/?term=Long-acting+beta2-agonists+in+asthma%3A+an+overview+of+Cochrane+systematic+reviews

21. Wikipedia. "Spirometry." (2016).
https://en.wikipedia.org/wiki/Spirometry

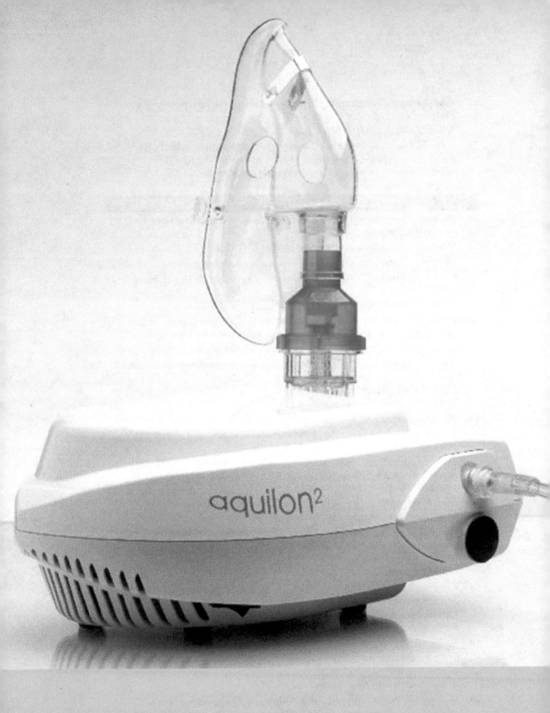

PART FOUR

Assessing, Treating, and Monitoring Asthma

In Part Three, we discussed how your physician makes a diagnosis of asthma. Part Four focuses on determining asthma severity, developing an asthma treatment plan, and monitoring the control of asthmatic symptoms. Asthma medications will be described in detail including new medications under development.

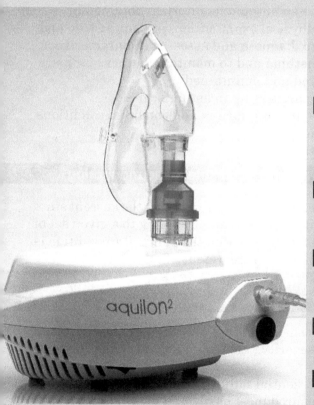

Source: Wikipedia

What are the basic principles for asthma assessment and monitoring according to the NAEPP (EPR-3)?

54. What are the four components of asthma care?

The National Asthma Education and Prevention Program (NAEPP) submitted "Expert Panel Report 3: Guidelines for the Diagnosis and Management of Asthma" (EPR-3) that organizes recommendations for asthma care around four components considered essential to effective asthma management:

- Measures of assessment and monitoring, obtained by objective tests, physical examination, patient history and patient report, to diagnose and assess the characteristics and severity of asthma and to monitor whether asthma control is achieved and maintained.
- Education for a partnership in asthma care.
- Control of environmental factors and comorbid conditions that affect asthma.
- Pharmacologic therapy.

55. What is meant by asthma assessment and monitoring?

Asthma assessment refers to a determination of the current state of the asthmatic condition of a patient according to a given set of criteria. Monitoring refers to how well the asthmatic condition is being controlled by following a treatment plan.

56. In what ways are asthma assessment and monitoring linked to each other?

The functions of assessment and monitoring are closely linked to the concepts of severity, control, and responsiveness to treatment:

- — Severity: the essential nature of the disease process. Severity is measured most easily and directly in a patient not receiving long-term control therapy.

— Control: the degree to which the manifestations of asthma (symptoms, functional impairments, and risks of untoward events) are minimized and the goals of therapy are met.

— Responsiveness: the ease with which asthma control is achieved by therapy.
Both severity and control include the fields of current impairment and future risk:

— Impairment: frequency and intensity of symptoms and limitations in daily activities the patient is experiencing or has recently experienced.

— Risk: the likelihood of either asthma exacerbations, progressive decline in lung function (or, for children, reduced lung growth), or risk of adverse effects from medication.
The concepts of severity and control are used as follows for managing asthma:

— During a patient's initial presentation, if the patient is not currently taking long-term control medication, asthma severity is assessed to guide clinical decisions on the appropriate medication and other therapeutic interventions.

— Once therapy is initiated, the emphasis for clinical management changes to assessing asthma control. Decisions to either maintain or adjust therapy will be based on the level of asthma control.

Diagnosing a patient as having asthma is only the first step in reducing the symptoms, functional limitations, impairment in quality of life, and risk of adverse events that are associated with the disease. The ultimate goal of treatment is to enable a patient to live with none of these manifestations of asthma, and an initial assessment of the severity of the disease allows an estimate of the type and intensity of treatment needed. Responsiveness to asthma treatment is variable; therefore, to achieve the goals of therapy, follow-up assessment must be made, and treatment should be adjusted accordingly. Even patients who have asthma that is well controlled at the time of a clinical assessment must be monitored over time, for the processes underlying asthma can vary in intensity over time, and treatment should be adjusted accordingly.

An important point linking asthma severity, control, and responsiveness is that the goals are identical for all levels of baseline asthma severity. A patient who has severe persistent asthma compared to a patient who has mild persistent asthma, or a patient who is less responsive to therapy may require more intensive intervention to achieve well-controlled asthma; however, the goals are the same: in well-controlled asthma, the manifestations of asthma are minimized by therapeutic intervention.

Although the severity of disease is most accurately assessed in patients before initiating long-term control medication, many patients are already receiving treatment when first seen by a new health care provider. In such cases, severity can be inferred from the least amount of treatment required to maintain control. This approach presumes that the severity of asthma is closely related to its responsiveness to treatment. Although this assumption may not be true for all forms of asthma and all treatments, it does focus attention on what is important in managing patients who have asthma: achieving a satisfactory level of control.

Both asthma severity and asthma control can be broken down into two domains: impairment and risk. Impairment is an assessment of the frequency and intensity of symptoms and functional limitations that a patient is experiencing or has recently experienced. Risk is an estimate of the likelihood of either asthma exacerbations or of progressive loss of pulmonary function over time.

– An assessment of the impairment domain for determining the severity of disease (in patients on no long-term control treatment before treatment is initiated) or the level of control (after treatment is selected) usually can be brought out by careful, directed history and lung function measurement.

– Assessment of the risk domain—that is, of adverse events in the future, especially of exacerbations and of progressive, irreversible loss of pulmonary function—is more problematic. Some assessment of the risk of exacerbations can be inferred from the medical history. Patients who have had exacerbations requiring emergency department visits, hospitalization, or intensive care unit (ICU) admission, especially in the past year, have a great risk of exacerbations in the future. Conversely, the achievement of good control of asthma symptoms and airflow obstruction from treatment with an inhaled corticosteroid (ICS) lowers the risk of asthma exacerbations in the future. It is not known, however, whether the minimum treatment to control symptoms will reduce the risk of exacerbations. Some patients who have few current symptoms or impairment of quality of life may still be at grave risk of severe, even life-threatening exacerbations. Finally, little is known about the prevalence of a heightened risk of progressive loss of pulmonary function among patients who have asthma or whether any current treatment can prevent it.

Assessment of response to therapy is important, but there is an inconsistency about the definition and measurement of "response." In general, response to therapy describes the ease with which adequate control is achieved by therapy.

The EPR-3 classification tables for asthma severity

57. What is the current classification of asthma severity?

The EPR-3 guideline classifies asthma into four groups: intermittent, persistent-mild, persistent-moderate, and persistent-severe. This classification can be used as a guide to develop a treatment plan.

58. What is the classification of a person's asthma according to current impairment and future risk?

Impairment refers to the limitations in activity or the degree of symptoms the patient experiences on a day-to-day basis. The components of impairment evaluation include daytime symptoms, nighttime awakenings, frequency of beta-agonist medication use for symptom relief, and difficulty with normal activities because of symptoms.

Future risk refers to the likelihood of either asthma exacerbations, progressive decline in lung function (or, for children, reduced lung growth), or risk of adverse effects from medication.

59. What are the classification levels of asthma severity?

The classification of level of asthma severity is determined by an assessment of current impairment and future risk.

The classification of level of control of asthma is also determined by an assessment of impairment and risk. The EPR-3 classification of asthma control consists of well controlled, not well controlled, and very poorly controlled.

It is important to understand that the following classification categories are guidelines for the physician to use in assessing a patient's asthma severity or control. There are many factors to take into consideration in evaluating a patient's condition. Some physicians prefer to use their own criteria to assess their patient's degree of asthma severity and control.

Interpretation of symbols:
< means less than
≤ means less than or equal to
> means greater than
≥ means greater than or equal to

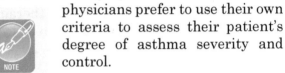

The following three tables classify people in three categories: children 0–4 years of age, children 5–11 years of age, and children 12 years of age and above and adults. These age groups have characteristics in common regarding the asthmatic condition.

Table 9.1 Assessment of asthma severity in children 0–4 years of age

Components of Severity		Classification of Asthma Severity (0–4 years of age)			
		Intermittent	Persistent		
			Mild	Moderate	Severe
Impairment	Symptoms	≤ 2 days/week	> 2 days/week but not daily	Daily	Throughout the day
	Nighttime awakenings	0	> 2 days/week but not daily	3–4 × /month	<1 × /week
	Short-acting beta$_2$-agonist* use for symptom control	≤ 2 days/week	> 2 days/week but not daily	Daily	Several times per day
	Interference with normal activity	None	Minor Limitation	Some limitation	Extremely limited

Components of Severity		Classification of Asthma Severity (0–4 years of age)			
		Intermittent	Persistent		
			Mild	Moderate	Severe
Risk	Exacerbations requiring oral systemic corticosteroids**	0–1 /year	≥ 2 exacerbations requiring oral systemic corticosteroids, or ≥ 4 wheezing episodes/ year lasting > 1 day		

*Beta$_2$-agonists are asthma drugs discussed in Chapter 10.
**Corticosteroids are asthma drugs discussed in Chapter 10.
Very young children are not given lung function tests because they are not able to follow instructions necessary to conduct the test. Note the increasing frequency of symptoms and nighttime awakenings as asthma progresses from intermittent to persistent severe. β-agonists are asthma medications that are used to provide quick relief of asthmatic symptoms. Quick relief indicates reversibility of symptoms. Some patients do not show relief of asthma symptoms until they have received 2–3 weeks of oral systemic corticosteroid treatments. These medications will be discussed later in the book.

Table 9.2 Assessment of asthma severity in children 5–11 years of age

Components of Severity		Classification of Asthma Severity (5–11 years of age)			
		Intermittent	Persistent		
			Mild	Moderate	Severe
Impairment	Symptoms	≤ 2 days/ week	> 2 days/ week but not daily	Daily	Throughout the day
	Nighttime awakenings	≤ 2 × /month	3–4 × /month	> 1 × /week but not nightly	Often 7×/ week
	Short-acting beta$_2$- agonist use for symptom relief	≤ 2 days/ week	> 2 days/ week but not daily	Daily	Several times per day
	Interference with normal activity	None	Minor limitation	Some limitation	Extremely limited
	Lung function	> 80% of normal	> 80% of normal	60–80% of normal	< 60% of normal
Risk	Exacerbations requiring oral systemic corticoster-oids	0–1/year	≥ 2/year		

Notes: The lung function tests FEV$_1$ and FVC were discussed in Question 49. FEV$_1$ is the volume of air expired in 1 second. The FEV$_1$ values are shown as percentages of predicted values. A decrease in FEV$_1$ values indicates the asthma is becoming more severe. FVC is forced vital capacity or the maximum volume of air exhaled after taking in as deep a breath as possible. The ratio FEV$_1$/FVC, when calculated as a percentage, is considered to be a more sensitive measure of pulmonary obstruction than FEV$_1$ alone. This improved sensitivity is borne out in the table.

Table 9.3 Assessment of asthma severity in youths ≥ 12 years of age and adults

Components of Severity		Classification of Asthma Severity ≥ 12 Years of Age			
				Persistent	
		Intermittent	Mild	Moderate	Severe
Impairment	Symptoms	≤ 2 days/ week	> 2 days/ week but not daily	Daily	Throughout the day
	Nighttime awakenings	≤ 2×/month	3–4 × /month	>1×/week but not nightly	Often 7×/ week
	Short-acting beta$_2$- agonist use for symptom control	≤ 2 days/ week	>2 days/ week but not daily, and not more than 1× on any day	Daily	Several times per day
	Interference with normal activity	None	Minor limitation	Some limitation	Extremely limited
	Lung function	> 80% of normal	> 80% of normal	Between 60 and 80% of normal	<60% of normal
Risk	Exacerbations requiring oral systemic corticosteroids	0–1/year	≥ 2/year Frequency and severity may fluctuate over time for patients in any severity category		

60. Why does the use of short-acting bronchodilators indicate asthma severity?

Short-acting bronchodilators are beta$_2$-agonist drugs that provide rapid, short-term relief of symptoms. These drugs are used to demonstrate reversibility of symptoms (symptoms go away) in the classification of asthma severity. As asthma becomes more severe, a person requires more frequent use of beta-agonist drugs.

The EPR-3 guidelines for asthma control

61. What are the key points in the assessment of asthma control?

- The goals of therapy are to achieve asthma control by:
  - Reducing impairment:
    - Prevent chronic and troublesome symptoms (e.g., coughing or breathlessness in the daytime, in the night, or after exertion)
    - Require infrequent use ($\leq$2 days a week) of inhaled short-acting beta$_2$-agonists for quick relief of symptoms
    - Maintain near "normal" pulmonary function
    - Maintain normal activity levels (including exercise and other physical activity and attendance at work or school)
    - Meet patients' and families' expectations of and satisfaction with asthma care
  - Reducing risk:
    - Prevent recurrent exacerbations of asthma and minimize the need for emergency department visits or hospitalizations
    - Prevent progressive loss of lung function; for children, prevent reduced lung growth
    - Provide optimal pharmacotherapy with minimal or no adverse effects
- Periodic assessments (at 1- to 6-month intervals) and ongoing monitoring of asthma control are recommended to determine if the goals of therapy are being met and if adjustments in therapy are needed. Measurements of the following are recommended:
  - Signs and symptoms of asthma
  - Pulmonary function
  - Quality of life/functional status
  - History of asthma exacerbations
  - Pharmacotherapy (checking for adherence to therapy and potential side effects from medication)
  - Patient–provider communication and patient satisfaction

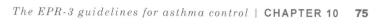

- Clinician assessment and patient self-assessment are the primary methods for monitoring asthma.
- The following frequencies for spirometry tests are recommended: (1) at the time of initial assessment, (2) after treatment is initiated and symptoms and PEF (peak expiratory flow measurements) have stabilized, (3) during periods of progressive or prolonged loss of asthma control, and (4) at least every 1–2 years.
- Use of minimally invasive markers ("biomarkers") to monitor asthma control and guide treatment decisions for therapy should be considered.
- Provide to all patients a written asthma action plan based on signs and symptoms and peak expiratory flow measurements; written action plans are particularly recommended for patients who have moderate or severe persistent asthma, a history of severe exacerbations, or poorly controlled asthma.
- Self-monitoring by the patient is important for effective self-management of asthma.
- Patients should be taught to recognize symptom patterns indicating inadequate asthma control and the need for additional therapy.
- Consider peak flow monitoring for patients who have moderate or severe persistent asthma, patients who have a history of severe exacerbations, and patients who poorly perceive airflow obstruction and worsening asthma.

62. What seven areas should be monitored to assess asthma control?

- Monitor signs and symptoms of asthma
- Monitor pulmonary function by:
  - Spirometry
  - Peak flow monitoring
- Monitor quality of life
- Monitor history of asthma exacerbations
- Monitor pharmacotherapy for adherence and potential side effects
- Monitor patient–provider communication and patient satisfaction
- Monitor asthma control with minimally invasive markers and pharmacogenetics (of increasing interest, but needs further evaluation)

Asthma control can be classified as well controlled, not well controlled, or very poorly controlled. The components of control are categorized under impairment and risk (similar to classifications of asthma severity). The following tables illustrate how asthma control is classified:

Table 10.1. Assessment of asthma control in children 0–4 years of age

Components of Control		Classification of Asthma Control (Children 0–4 Years of Age)		
		Well Controlled	Not Well Controlled	Very Poorly Controlled
Impairment	Symptoms	≤2 days/week	> 2 days/week	Throughout the day
	Nighttime awakenings	≤1×/month	> 1×/month	> 1×/week
	Interference with normal activity	None	Some limitation	Extremely limited
	Short-acting beta$_2$-agonist use for symptom relief	≤ 2 days/week	> 2 days/week	Several times per day
Risk	Exacerbations requiring oral systemic corticosteroids	0–1/year	2–3/year	> 3/year
	Adverse effects due to treatments	Side effects due to medications can vary from none to very troublesome and worrisome. The intensity of side effects does not relate to specific levels of control.		

Table 10.2. Assessment of asthma control in children 5–11 years of age

Components of Control		Classification of Asthma Control (Children 5–11 Years of Age)		
		Well Controlled	Not Well Controlled	Very Poorly Controlled
Impairment	Symptoms	≤ 2 days/week but not more than once on each day	> 2 days/week or multiple times on ≤ 2 days/week	Throughout the day
	Nighttime awakenings	≤ 1×/month	≥ 2×/month	≥ 2×/week
	Interference with normal activity	None	Some limitation	Extremely limited
	Short-acting beta$_2$-agonist use for symptom control	≤ 2 days/week	>2 days/week	Several times per day
	Lung function	> 80% of normal	60–80% of normal	< 60% of normal
Risk	Exacerbations requiring oral systemic corticosteroids	0–1/year	≥ 2/year	
	Reduction in lung growth	Evaluation requires long-term follow-up		
	Adverse effects due to treatments	Side effects due to medications can vary from none to very troublesome and worrisome. The intensity of side effects does not relate to specific levels of control.		

Table 10.3. Assessing asthma control in youths ≥12 years of age and adults

Components of Control		Classification of Asthma Control (Youths ≥12 Years of Age and Adults)		
		Well Controlled	Not wellControlled	Very Poorly Controlled
Impairment	Symptoms	≤ 2 days/week	> 2 days/week	Throughout the day
	Nighttime awakening	≤ 2×/month	1–3×/week	≥ 4×/week
	Interference with normal activity	None	Some limitation	Extremely limited
	Short-acting beta$_2$-agonist use for symptom control	≤ 2 days/week	> 2 days/week	Several times per day
	Lung function	>80 % of normal	60–80% of normal	<60% of normal
Risk	Exacerbations	0–1/year	≥ 2/year	
	Progressive loss of lung function	Evaluation requires long-term follow-up care		
	Adverse effects due to treatments	Side effects due to medications can vary from none to very troublesome and worrisome. The intensity of side effects does not relate to specific levels of control.		

Medications for asthma

CHAPTER 11

ON THE WEB

The National Heart, Lung, and Blood Institute prepared an excellent video on research on new treatments for severe asthma. Visit: https://www.nhlbi.nih.gov/health/health-topics/topics/asthma/

64. What are the two main categories of asthma medications?

- Long-term control medications used to achieve and maintain control of persistent asthma
- Quick-relief medications taken to provide prompt reversal of acute airflow obstruction and relief of accompanying bronchoconstriction

Patients who have persistent asthma require both classes of medications.

65. What is your doctor's overall strategy for prescribing asthma medications?

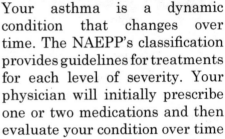

Long-term control medications are also known as long-term preventive, controller, or maintenance medications. Quick relief medications are also known as reliever or rescue medications.

Your asthma is a dynamic condition that changes over time. The NAEPP's classification provides guidelines for treatments for each level of severity. Your physician will initially prescribe one or two medications and then evaluate your condition over time to see how well your asthma is being controlled. Your physician may very well change your medications, or increase or decrease the medication dosages, depending on how well your asthma is being controlled.

66. Why are aerosols the best way to deliver asthma medications?

Aerosols deliver medications in vapor form directly into the air passages using metered dose inhalers, dry powder inhalers, and nebulizers. There are several advantages in delivering drugs by aerosols compared to the oral route (swallowing pills or liquids):

- The medications are delivered at high concentrations directly to the airways where they are needed.
- Very little of the medications are absorbed into the systemic circulation (the rest of the body) where they could cause adverse side effects.
- Symptoms are relieved faster with the use of inhalers and nebulizers than with the use of oral products (particularly important during episodes of exacerbation).

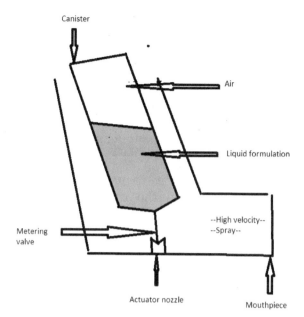

Canister

Air

Liquid formulation

--High velocity--
--Spray--

Metering
valve

Actuator nozzle

Mouthpiece

◀ **Figure 11.1**
Diagram of a metered dose inhaler

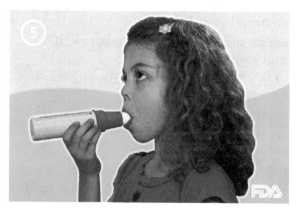

◀ **Figure 11.2**
Metered dose inhaler in action
Credit : U.S. Food & Drug Administration

67. How does a metered dose inhaler work?

A metered dose inhaler (MDI) consists of a canister of liquid medication under pressure with a propellant that fits in a plastic sleeve that connects to a mouthpiece (see Figure 11.1). As the patient presses down on the canister, the liquid medication passes through a metering valve and actuator nozzle. The metering valve is calibrated to dispense the correct amount of medication. The medication is converted into a high-velocity spray that the patient then inhales into the airways.

The type of propellant used in inhalers has changed as a result of the 1997 Montreal Protocol. The Protocol mandated the phase out of fluorocarbon use in propellants to protect the ozone layer in the atmosphere. Current inhalers use hydrofluroalkane as a propellant. This new propellant is more effective as it produces an aerosol with a smaller particle size that enters the airways more efficiently.

68. How do you use a metered dose inhaler?

The following are general steps for how to use and clean a metered-dose inhaler. Be sure to read the instructions that come with your inhaler. Ask your doctor, pharmacist, or other health care professional (such as nurse practitioner, physician assistant, nurse, respiratory therapist, or asthma educator) to show you how to use your inhaler. Review your technique at each follow-up visit.

1. Take off the cap. Shake the inhaler. Prime (spray or pump) the inhaler as needed according to manufacturer's instructions (each brand is different).
2. If you use a spacer or valved holding chamber (VHC), remove the cap and look into the mouthpiece to make sure nothing is in it. Place the inhaler in the rubber ring on the end of the spacer/VHC.
3. Stand up or sit up straight.
4. Take in a deep breath. Tilt head back slightly and blow out completely to empty your lungs.
5. Place the mouthpiece of the inhaler or spacer/VHC in your mouth and close your lips around it to form a tight seal.
6. As you start to breathe in, press down firmly on the top of the medicine canister to release one "puff" (dose) of medicine. Breathe in slowly (gently) and as deeply as you can for 3–5 seconds.
7. Hold your breath and count to 10.
8. Take the inhaler or spacer/VHC out of your mouth. Breathe out slowly.
9. If you are supposed to take two puffs of medicine per dose, wait 1 minute and repeat steps 3 through 8.
10. If using an inhaled corticosteroid, rinse out your mouth with water and spit it out. Rinsing will help to prevent an infection in the mouth.

Table 11.1. Issues using MDIs

Available Drugs for Use	Patient Age	Optimal Technique	Therapeutic Issues
Beta₂-agonists Corticosteroids Cromolyn sodium Anticholinergics	≥ 5 years old (< 5 with spacer or valved holding chamber [VHC] mask)	Actuation during a slow (30 L/min or 3–5 seconds) deep inhalation, followed by 10-second breath hold	Slow inhalation and coordination of actuation during inhalation may be difficult, particularly in young children and elderly
			Patients may incorrectly stop inhalation at actuation
			Deposition of 50–80% of actuated dose in the oropharynx (part of the throat that is at the back of the mouth)
			Mouth washing and spitting is effective in reducing the amount of drug swallowed and absorbed systemically
			Lung delivery under ideal conditions varies significantly between MDIs due to differences in formulation (suspension versus solution), and valve design

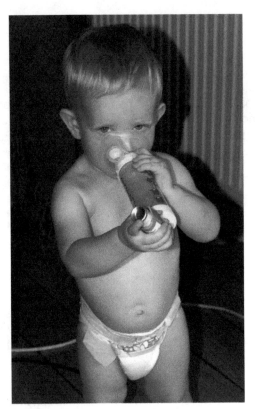

▲ **Figure 11.3**
Baby using inhaler, spacer, and mask
Credit: Phyllis Buchanan
Creative Commons

Use of a face mask with infants allows asthma medications to be delivered via MDIs. Infants typically inhale less medication into the lungs. Small particle aerosols may provide better lung deposition.

69. How can spacers be beneficial?

Spacers (also known as holding chambers) are hollow tubes that fit over the mouthpiece of the inhaler. Spacers have their mouthpiece at the other end. Spacers were designed to overcome problems that patients commonly experience when administering medication via an MDI. Spacers were developed in direct response to patient problems with MDI technique, particularly, poor coordination between pressing down on the canister and inhalation, and side-effects arising from deposition of medication in the mouth and pharynx. Spacers permit the aerosol plume from the inhaler to expand and slow down, turning it into a very fine mist instead of a high-velocity spray. The fine drug particles are more likely to be carried deep into the airways where they are needed instead of remaining in the mouth or pharynx.

Spacers may help the delivery of medications as they allow you to inhale your dose over several breaths. Spacers can be particularly useful for young children who may have difficulty in coordinating breathing with an inhaler. Young children are typically fitted with a mask as well as the mouthpiece.

Table 11.2. Issues using spacers or valved holding chambers (VHCs)

Drugs Used	Patient Age	Optimal Technique	Therapeutic Issues
Beta$_2$-agonists Corticosteroids Cromolyn sodium Anticholinergics (same as MDIs)	≥ 4 years old	Slow (30 L/min or 3–5 seconds) deep inhalation, followed by 10-second breath hold immediately following actuation. Actuate only once into spacer/VHC per inhalation Rinse plastic VHCs once a month with low concentration of liquid household dishwashing detergent (1:5,000 or 1–2 drops per cup of water) and let drip dry	Indicated for patients who have difficulty performing adequate MDI technique May be bulky Simple tubes do not obviate coordinating actuation and inhalation The VHCs are preferred Spacers and/or VHCs decrease oropharyngeal deposition and thus decrease risk of topical side effects (e.g., thrush) Spacers will also reduce the potential systemic availability of ICSs with higher oral absorption

(Contd.)

Drugs Used	Patient Age	Optimal Technique	Therapeutic Issues
			However, spacer/VHCs may increase the systemic availability of ICSs that are poorly absorbed orally by enhancing delivery to lungs
			Use antistatic VHCs or rinse plastic nonantistatic VHCs with dilute household detergents to enhance delivery to lungs and efficacy
			As effective as nebulizer for delivering SABAs and anticholinergics in mild to moderate exacerbations
	< 4 years old VHC with face mask	If face mask is used, it should have a tight fit and allow 3–5 inhalations per actuation	Face mask allows MDIs to be used with small children
			However, the use of a face mask reduces delivery to the lungs by 50%
			The VHC improves lung delivery and response in patients who have poor MDI technique

Use of a face mask with infants allows asthma medications to be delivered via MDIs. Infants typically inhale less medication into the lungs. Small particle aerosols may provide better lung deposition.

70. What are common mistakes in using metered-dose inhalers?

Using metered-dose inhalers require multiple steps, and studies have shown that patients make at least one mistake as much as 90% of the time. As a result, only about 7% to 40% of drugs are delivered to the lungs. Follow-up visits with your doctor are important as physicians realize that their patients can become lax over time in metered-dose inhaler use. The following are the most common errors in metered-dose inhaler use:

- Failing to shake the inhaler well. Shaking is recommended before each puff, but many patients only shake before the first puff.
- Orientation. Inhalers should be held upright for correct delivery of medicine.
- Exhibiting poor coordination. Patients fail to press down on the canister and inhale simultaneously. Using spacers may help people with coordination problems.
- Breathing in too quickly. Patients should breath in slowly and deeply.
- Holding their breath. Patients fail to hold their breath for 5-10 seconds after breathing in to allow time for the medication to settle in their lungs.
- Spacing. Many patients fail to wait 15-30 seconds before taking the next puff.

For an excellent discussion and video on the proper use of metered-dose inhalers, visit: https://www.wsj.com/articles/many-asthma-patients-use-their-inhalers-incorrectly-research-shows-1488822193

71. What are breath-actuated metered dose inhalers?

Breath-actuated MDIs are a different form of MDI. Breath actuated MDIs were developed to overcome the problem of poor coordination of canister actuation and inspiration that some patients have, especially the elderly. With breath-actuated MDIs, medications are brought into the lungs by inspiration rather than by a propellant.

To use, the patient forms a good seal around the mouthpiece and inhales slowly. The breathing in and breath-hold are the same as with a regular MDI. Getting the right speed of inhalation—some patients find it difficult to inhale slowly—and the fact that not all medications are available for breath-actuated MDIs are disadvantages.

Table 11.3. Issues using breath-actuated MDIs

Drugs Available	Patient Age	Optimal Technique	Therapeutic Issues
Only beta$_2$-agonist	≥ 5 years old	Tight seal around mouthpiece and slightly more rapid inhalation than standard MDI followed by 10-second breath hold.	May be particularly useful for patients unable to coordinate inhalation and actuation.
			May also be useful for elderly patients Patients may incorrectly stop inhalation at actuation
			Cannot be used with currently available spacer/valved-holding chamber (VHC) devices

72. What are valved holding chambers (VHCs)?

A valved holding chamber is a type of spacer that includes a one-way valve at the mouthpiece. The one-way valve stops you from accidentally exhaling into the tube. Thus, patients—either very young children or infants or those who for some other reason are unable to cooperate—can breathe normally and have someone else actuate the device without loss of the actuated dose and obviating the need for coordinating actuation and inhalation.

Valved holding chambers have the following benefits:
- Lessen the need to precisely time inhalation with activation and pumping of the canister
- Enhances delivery of medication into the airways
- Decreases deposition of medicine in the throat and tongue lessening the risk of side effects such as cough, hoarseness, fungus infections, and throat irritations

The use of VHCs may result in inconsistent medication delivery due to the following:
- Electrostatic charges resulting from interaction between the aerosol and interior surfaces of the VHC. To minimize this effect, prewash the VHC with an ionic detergent

- Incorrect operation of inhalation and exhalation valves
- The fit of the facemask, when used, is not tight to the face

73. When are dry powder inhalers advantageous to use?

Dry powder inhalers (DPIs) were developed as an alternative delivery device for asthma medications. DPIs can administer predetermined doses of corticosteroids or long-acting bronchodilators in dry powder form singly or in combination. This type of inhaler requires an adequate inspiratory flow rate for drug delivery, as it does not include a propellant. Because of this inspiratory flow rate requirement, most DPIs are not appropriate for treatment of exacerbations or for young children under 5 years of age.

Using a DPI requires you to take a controlled, deep breath so that the medication in the form of a very fine powder reaches deeply in the airways. For people who have difficulty in coordinating the steps required in using a metered dose inhaler, a DPI may be a better alternative.

There are many manufacturers of DPIs, each with unique features requiring different instructions for use. The degree of resistance to inspiratory flow required to aerosolize the medication varies with each DPI. Diskus© is a low-resistance device and thus is suitable for treatment of children and those with decreased lung function. Other DPIs require a higher inspiratory flow rate to aerosolize an equivalent drug dose.

74. How do you use a dry powder inhaler?

The following are general steps for how to use and clean a dry powder inhaler. Be sure to read the instructions that come with your inhaler.

1. Remove cap and hold inhaler upright (like a rocket). A Discus© inhaler has a unique shape (like a flying saucer). This inhaler should be held flat.
2. Load a dose of medicine according to manufacturer's instructions (each brand of inhaler is different; you may have to prime the inhaler the first time you use it). Do not shake the inhaler.
3. Stand up or sit up straight.
4. Take a deep breath in and blow out completely to empty your lungs. Do not blow into the inhaler.

5. Place the mouthpiece of the inhaler in your mouth and close your lips around it to form a tight seal.

6. Take a fast, deep, forceful breath in through your mouth.

7. Hold your breath and count to 10.

8. Take the inhaler out of your mouth. Breathe out slowly, facing away from the inhaler.

9. If you are supposed to take more than one inhalation of medicine per dose, wait 1 minute and repeat steps 2 through 8.

10. When you finish, put the cover back on the inhaler or slide the cover closed. Store the inhaler in a cool, dry place (not in the bathroom).

11. If using an inhaled corticosteroid, rinse out your mouth with water and spit it out. Rinsing helps to prevent an infection in the mouth.

Table 11.4. Issues using dry powder inhalers

Drugs Available	Patient Age	Optimal Technique	Therapeutic Issues
Beta$_2$-agonists Corticosteroids Anticholinergics	≥ 4 years old	Rapid (60 L/min or 1–2 seconds), deep inhalation. Minimally effective inspiratory flow is device dependent Most children < 4 years of age may not generate sufficient inspiratory flow to activate the inhaler	The dose is lost if the patient exhales through device after actuating Delivery may be greater or lesser than MDI, depending on device and technique Delivery is more flow dependent in devices with highest internal resistance Rapid inhalation promotes greater deposition in larger central airways

Drugs Available	Patient Age	Optimal Technique	Therapeutic Issues
			Mouth washing and spitting is effective in reducing amount of drug swallowed and absorbed

75. What are nebulizers?

Nebulizers convert liquid medications into an aerosol (mist), and come in two basic types, jet nebulizers and ultrasonic nebulizers. Jet nebulizers use an air compressor to bubble air or oxygen through a liquid containing the medication resulting in the formation of mist. Ultrasonic nebulizers use a high-frequency crystal to produce the aerosol. Most physicians prefer jet nebulizers as they produce more uniformly sized medicine particles for inhalation.

Nebulizers provide a vehicle for drug delivery to patients who are too ill or too young to use metered dose inhalers, as nebulizers do not need the coordination between hand movements and breathing that are necessary for inhaler use. Nebulizers come in home and portable devices. Home nebulizers are larger and must be plugged into an electrical outlet. Portable nebulizers run on batteries, and can be carried in a purse, briefcase, or backpack.

Recently, breath-actuated nebulizers (BANs) were developed as an improvement over standard jet nebulizers. Preliminary studies have shown that both patients and respiratory therapists have shown greater satisfaction with BANs. The use of BANs was associated with a shorter duration and lower occurrence of adverse asthma events. BANs are equipped with a one-way mouthpiece that creates aerosol only during the inspiratory phase.

76. How do you use a nebulizer?

The following are general steps for how to use and clean a nebulizer. Be sure to read the instructions that come with your nebulizer.

1. Wash hands well.

2. Put together the nebulizer machine, tubing, medicine cup, and mouthpiece or mask according to manufacturer's instructions.

3. Put the prescribed amount of medicine into the medicine cup. If your medicine comes in a premeasured capsule or vial, empty it into the cup.

4. Place the mouthpiece in your mouth and close your lips around it to form a tight seal. If your child uses a mask, make sure it fits snugly over your child's nose and mouth. Never hold the mouthpiece or mask away from the face.

5. Turn on the nebulizer machine. You should see a light mist coming from the back of the tube opposite the mouthpiece or the mask.

6. Take normal breaths through the mouth while the machine is on. Continue treatment until the medicine cup is empty or the mist stops, about 10 minutes.

7. Take the mouthpiece out of your mouth (or remove mask) and turn off the machine.

8. If using an inhaled corticosteroid, rinse mouth with water and spit it out. If using a mask, also wash the face.

How to clean and store a nebulizer

One disadvantage of a nebulizer over MDIs or DPIs is that they require more maintenance.

After each treatment:
- Wash hands well.
- Wash the medicine cup and mouthpiece or mask with warm water and mild soap. Do not wash the tubing.
- Rinse well and shake off excess water. Air dry parts on a paper towel. Once a week:
  Disinfect nebulizer parts to help kill any germs. Follow instructions for each nebulizer part listed in the package insert. Always remember:
- Do not wash or boil the tubing.
- Air dry parts on a paper towel.

Between uses:
- Store nebulizer parts in a dry, clean plastic storage bag. If the nebulizer is used by more than one person, keep each person's medicine cup, mouthpiece or mask, and

tubing in a separate, labeled bag to prevent the spread of germs.

- Wipe surface with a clean, damp cloth as needed. Cover nebulizer machine with a clean, dry cloth and store as manufacturer instructs.
- Replace medicine cup, mouthpiece, mask, tubing, filter, and other parts according to manufacturer's instructions or when they appear worn or damaged.

Table 11.5 Issues using nebulizers

Drugs Available	Patient Age	Optimal Technique	Therapeutic Issues
Beta$_2$-agonists Corticosteroids Cromolyn sodium Anticholinergics	Patients of any age who cannot use MDI with VHC and face mask	Slow tidal breathing with occasional deep breaths Tightly fitting face mask for those unable to use mouthpiece	Less dependent on patient's coordination and cooperation Delivery method of choice for cromolyn sodium in young children May be expensive; time consuming; bulky; output is dependent on device and operating parameters (fill volume, driving gas flow); internebulizer and intranebulizer output variances are significant Use of a face mask reduces delivery to lungs by 50%

Drugs Available	Patient Age	Optimal Technique	Therapeutic Issues
			Nebulizers are as effective as MDIs plus VHCs for delivering bronchodilators in the ED for mild to moderate exacerbations; data in severe exacerbations are limited
			Choice of delivery system is dependent on resources, availability, and clinical judgment of the clinician caring for the patient
			Potential for bacterial infections if not cleaned properly

77. How are medications categorized?

Medications for asthma are categorized into two general classes: long-term control medications used to achieve and maintain control of persistent asthma and quick-relief medications used to treat acute symptoms and exacerbations. We will discuss long-term medications first.

78. What are the long-term medications?

The NAEPP recommends that long-term control medications be taken daily on a long-term basis to achieve and maintain control of persistent asthma. The most effective long-term control medications are those that lessen the underlying inflammation that is characteristic of asthma. Anti-inflammatory medications reduce swelling and mucus production in the airways. Their use can lead to reduction in symptoms, improvement in airflow, reduction in airway hyperresponsiveness, prevention of exacerbations, and prevention of damage to the airway (remodeling). Long-term control medications include inhaled corticosteroids, inhaled long-acting bronchodilators, leukotriene modifiers, cromolyn, theophylline, and immumomodulators.

79. How do corticosteroids work?

Corticosteroids are also known as glucocorticosteroids, glucocorticoids, or just steroids. Steroid hormones, particularly cortisol, are produced naturally by the adrenal gland. Corticosteroid drugs are structurally related to these natural steroid hormones. The NAEPP concludes that inhaled corticosteroids are the most potent and consistently effective long-term medication for asthma. The broad action of inhaled corticoterids (ICSs) on the inflammatory process may account for their efficacy as preventive therapy.

The clinical effects of corticosteroids include:
- Reduction in severity of symptoms
- Improved pulmonary functioning
- Diminished airway hyperresponsiveness
- Prevention of exacerbations
- Reduction in periods of treatment with systemic corticosteroids
- Reduced instances of emergency room and hospitalization visits
- Deaths due to asthma
- Possibly the lessening of loss of lung function in adults

Inhaled medications are preferable for asthma since they deliver medication directly to the airways with minimal side effects. Inhaled corticosteroids begin to reduce inflammation after one week and reach their full effect by four weeks.

Corticosteroids work by inhibiting the activity of genes responsible for the synthesis of molecules active in the inflammatory process.

80. What are the inhaled corticosteroid medications?

Inhaled corticosteroids are used for long-term prevention of symptoms and suppression, control, and reversal of inflammation. They also reduce the need for oral corticosteroids. They block late reaction to allergens and reduce airway hyper responsiveness.

Possible adverse effects include cough, speech difficulty, or oral fungus infection (candidiasis).

Systemic corticosteroids (taken orally) are used to gain prompt control of inadequately controlled persistent asthma. They are also used for long-term prevention of symptoms in severe persistent asthma, including suppression, control, and reversal of inflammation. Systemic corticosteroids are used to control asthma exacerbations when bronchodilators fail to control symptoms. Since use of systemic corticosteroids can cause many adverse effects, they are only used as needed and withdrawn when symptoms are under control. Adverse effects of short-term use may include: reversible abnormalities in glucose metabolism, increased appetite, fluid retention, weight gain, mood alteration, hypertension, and peptic ulcer. Adverse effects of long-term use may include: adrenal gland malfunctioning, Cushing syndrome, growth suppression, thinning of the dermis skin layer, hypertension, diabetes cataracts, and muscle weakness.

Table 11.6. Inhaled corticosteroid medications

Generic name	Brand name	Use
Beclomethasone Propionate	QVAR Inhalation Aerosol	Control/prevent asthma age 5 or older
Budesonide	Pulmicort Flexhaler	Control/prevent asthma age 6 or older
	Pulmicort Respules	Control/prevent asthma age 12 months to 8 years
Ciclesonide	Alvesco Inhalation Aeorsol	Maintenance of asthma age 12 and older
Flunisolide	Aerobid	Age 6 and older
	Aerobid-M	Adult
	Aerospan	Control/prevent asthma Age 6–11 Age 12 or older

Fluticasone Propionate	Flovent HFA Inhalation aerosol Flovent Diskus	Control/prevent asthma age 4 and above
Mometasone	Asmanex Twisthaler 220 mcg	Control/prevent asthma age 12 and over
	Asmanex Twisthaler 110 mcg	Control/prevent asthma age 4–11
Mometazone furoate HFA	Asmanex HFA	Prevent/control asthma age 12 years and older
Triaminolone Acetonide	Asmacort Inhalation Aerosol	Control/prevent asthma Age 6–12 Adults
Methylprednisolone	Medrol Generic	Asthma exacerbation
Prednisolone	Orapred Prelone Generic Pediapred Orapred ODT	Asthma exacerbation
Prednisone	Generic	Asthma exacerbation

How do you determine which corticosteroid medicine is best for you? Corticosteroids could be judged by the amount of medication necessary to achieve desired effects; such as improvement in lung function, reduction in asthmatic symptoms and susceptibility to asthmatic attacks, and a decrease in bronchial sensitivity. In practice, it can be difficult to make direct comparisons among corticosteroid medicines due to the many variables involved.

The variables involved are as follows:
- Concentration of medicine per puff. Concentration is related to potency which is the dose or amount of medication needed to achieve a specific effect of a given intensity. The amount of medicine taken in with each

inhalation can vary greatly among the corticosteroids. Of course, the amount of medicine reaching the bronchial tubes is of primary importance.

- Type of delivery system. As we have discussed, patients differ in their ability to properly use metered dose inhalers, which can limit the amount of medication inhaled with each puff. Adding spacers or holding chambers can be beneficial to improve delivery of medicine. Dry powder inhalers have found to be more effective in delivering medication to the bronchial tubes.
- Side effects. When medicines are formulated with higher concentrations, fewer puffs are necessary to achieve the desired effects. Higher concentrations can mean less exposure of the medicine to the throat and pharynx leading to less absorption of the medicine into the general circulation.
- Cost. The cost of the medicine should relate to the amount needed to achieve the desirable effects.

Given the variables involved, most physicians consider the corticosteroid medications to be roughly equivalent. The medication given to the patient may be due to physician preference. The experience of the patient with using the drug is paramount; as long as the drug works well, it will most likely be continued.

81. What actions can you take to reduce side effects with inhaled corticosteroid use?

To reduce the potential for adverse effects, EPR-3 recommends the following measures:

- Spacers or valved holding chambers (VHCs) used with non-breath-activated MDIs can reduce local side effects. These devices can reduce the colonization of *oral candidiasis*, a fungal infection commonly known as thrush; dysphonia (voice impairment); and reflex cough and bronchospasm.
- Patients should rinse their mouths (rinse and spit) after inhalation.
- The lowest dose of ICS that maintains asthma control should be used. Consider factors that may be contributing to asthma severity, such as patient adherence to medications and inhaler technique or changes in

environmental factors before increasing the dose of ICS. Increasing doses of ICS is also associated with dysphonia.

- To achieve or maintain control of asthma, consider adding a LABA (long-acting beta$_2$ agonist) to a low or medium dose of ICS rather than using a higher dose of ICS.
- Monitor growth of children.
- In adult patients, consider supplements of calcium (1,000–1,500 mg per day) and vitamin D (400–800 units a day), particularly in perimenopausal women. Bone-sparing therapy (e.g., bisphosphonate), where appropriate, may be considered for patients on medium or high doses of ICS, particularly for those who are at risk of osteoporosis or who have low bone mineral density (BMD) scores by dual energy x-ray absorptiometry (or DEXA) scan. In children, age-appropriate dietary intake of calcium and exercise should be reviewed with the child's caregivers.
- The potential for adverse effects on linear growth from ICS appears to be dose dependent. In treatment of children who have mild or moderate persistent asthma, low- to medium-dose ICS therapy may be associated with a possible, but not predictable, adverse effect on linear growth. The clinical significance of this potential systemic effect has yet to be determined. High doses of ICS have greater potential for growth suppression.

82. When would systemic corticosteroids be used?

Systemic corticosteroids are given orally (as pills or liquid) or occasionally by injection. Systemic corticosteroids travel throughout the body before reaching the airway, in contrast to inhaled corticosteroids that are directed to the airways with minimum exposure to the rest of the body.

Oral systemic corticosteroids suppress, control, and reverse airway inflammation. Before the development of inhaled corticosteroids, the systemic route was the only way to administer corticosteroid medicines. After long-term use, side effects were very noticeable. These effects include adrenal suppression, growth suppression, skin (dermal) thinning, hypertension, Cushing syndrome, cataracts, and muscle weakness. Cushing syndrome is due to prolonged exposure of the body's tissue to high levels of cortisol, whether this cortisol is due to excessive secretions of the adrenal gland or from synthetic corticosteroids (medications).

EPR-3 recommends that chronic administration of oral systemic corticosteroids as a long-term control medication be used only for the most severe, difficult-to-control asthma because of well-documented risk for side effects.

EPR-3 recommends that, because the magnitude of adverse effects is often related to the dose, frequency of administration, and the duration of corticosteroid use, every consideration should be given to minimize systemic corticosteroid doses and maximize other modes of therapy. It is necessary, therefore, to monitor the development and progression of adverse effects and to take appropriate steps to minimize the risk and impact of adverse corticosteroid effects.

When systemic corticosteroids are used on a short-term basis, the risk of side effects is greatly reduced. As a result, these medications have found an important place as quick-relief medications. These uses will be discussed in Question 90.

83. What are leukotriene modifiers?

Leukotrienes are potent biochemical mediators—released from mast cells, eosinophils, and basophils—that contract airway smooth muscle, increase vascular permeability, increase mucus secretions, and attract and activate inflammatory cells in the airways of patients who have asthma (see Question 30). Leukotriene modifiers work by blocking the action of leukotrienes.

Three leukotriene modifiers—montelukast, zafirlukast, and zileuton—are available as oral tablets for the treatment of asthma. Only montelukast (for children as young as 1 year of age) and zafirlukast (for children as young as 7 years of age) are approved for use in children.

Leukotriene receptor antagonists (LTRAs) are an alternative, not preferred, treatment option for mild persistent asthma. LTRAs can also be used as adjunct (additional) therapy with ICS, but for youths ≥12 years of age and adults, they are not the preferred, adjunct therapy compared to the addition of long-acting β-agonists (LABAs).

5-lipoxygenase is an enzyme that catalyzes the formation of leukotrienes. A 5-lipoxygenase inhibitor, therefore, reduces the formation of leukotrienes. Zileuton is a 5-lipoxygenase inhibitor used as an alternative treatment option but is less desirable than LTRAs. Patients who have moderate asthma treated with zileuton experience fewer exacerbations requiring oral systemic corticosteroids, thus suggesting anti-inflammatory action. Zileuton is capable of lessening bronchoconstriction from exercise and aspirin in aspirin-sensitive individuals. Zileuton has two main disadvantages: it exhibits liver toxicity and breaks down rapidly in the body requiring several daily doses.

84. What are cromolyn sodium and nedocromil?

Cromolyn and nedocromil are grouped together in a class of molecules known as chromones and have similar anti-inflammatory actions. In Question 32 (and Figure 4.1) we discussed the role of mast cells in releasing chemical messengers called histamine and leukotrienes that cause symptoms of asthma. Cromolyn and nedocromil work by preventing the release of these chemicals thereby reducing inflammation. They have gained use as alternative medications for the treatment of mild persistent asthma. They are considered alternative medications since they are less effective than inhaled corticosteroids. Using cromolyn or nedocromil can result in a lower incidence of side effects compared with the use of inhaled corticosteroids. They can also be used as preventive treatment before exercise or unavoidable exposure to known allergens.

The two medications are equally effective against allergen exposure, although nedocromil appears to be more potent than cromolyn in inhibiting bronchospasm provoked by exercise, by cold, dry air, and by bradykinin aerosol. EPR-3 has concluded that cromolyn could be considered as an alternative treatment for persistent asthma for children of all ages and nedocromil for children ≥5 years of age.

Cromolyn oral inhalation comes as a solution (liquid) to inhale by mouth using a nebulizer. When the nebulizer is used to prevent symptoms of asthma, it is usually used four times a day. When the nebulizer is used to prevent breathing difficulty caused by exercise, cold and dry air, or by inhaling a substance (trigger), it is usually used 10 to 15 minutes before exercise or before you come into contact with the asthma trigger. Follow the directions on your prescription label carefully, and ask your doctor or pharmacist to explain any part you do not understand. Use cromolyn exactly as directed. Do not use more or less of it or use it more often than prescribed by your doctor.

Cromolyn controls asthma but does not cure it. Your symptoms may improve soon after you begin using cromolyn, but it may take up to 4 weeks before you feel the full benefit of the medication. You should use it regularly for it to be effective. If your symptoms have not improved after 4 weeks, tell your doctor. Continue to use cromolyn even if you feel well. Do not stop using cromolyn without talking to your doctor.

Cromolyn oral inhalation helps to prevent excerbations, but will not stop an exacerbation that has already started. Your doctor will prescribe a short-acting inhaler to use during excerbations.

Before you use cromolyn inhalation for the first time, read the written instructions that come with the nebulizer. Ask your doctor, pharmacist, or respiratory therapist to show you how to use it. Practice using the nebulizer while he or she watches.

85. What are immunomodulators?

Immunotherapy is the "treatment of disease by inducing, enhancing, or suppressing an immune response," while immunomodulators are the active agents of immunotherapy. Immunomodulators are medications from natural or synthetic substances that help regulate or normalize an immune system that is out of balance. Asthma is notable for being an inflammatory process characterized by an abnormally increased immune response in the airways. Immunomodulators treat asthma by suppressing the immune system.

86. When should immunomodulators be used to treat asthma?

Although inhaled corticosteroids have proven to be very effective in controlling asthma, an estimated 30%–35% of patients have a poor or no response to these medicines. Immunotherapy has been introduced as a means of treating these patients, often in combination with other medicines. Several immunomodulators based on monoclonal antibody technology are now on the market and are being used to treat patients.

Omalizumab is a humanized monoclonal antibody produced in the laboratory by immunizing mice with human IgE antibody. Omalizumab recognizes and binds to IgE antibody produced in the body, thereby reducing the inflammation of allergic asthma.

NOTE Monoclonal antibodies are antibodies that are made by identical immune cells that are all clones (copies) of a unique parent cell. Each type of monoclonal antibody binds to a specific antigen.

Omalizumab is used as supporting therapy for patients ≥12 years of age who have allergies and severe persistent asthma. A small number of patients may experience anaphylactic shock as a side effect.

Mepolizumab is a humanized monoclonal antibody used to treat patients who have frequent exacerbations despite continuous treatment with high-dose inhaled glucocorticoids with or without oral corticosteroids. It recognizes and blocks interleukin-5, a signaling protein of the immune system. Mepolizumab is given either intravenously or subcutaneously (under the skin).

The most common side effects of mepolizumab include: headache, injection site reactions (pain, redness, swelling, itching, or a burning feeling at the injection site), back pain, and weakness (fatigue).

Reslizumab is a humanized monoclonal antibody against human interleukin-5. Reslizumab binds to interleukin-5, thereby reducing the activity of human eosinophils.

Reslizumab is used for supporting maintenance treatment of patients 18 years of age or over. It is given by intravenous infusion. Side effects include pain in the mouth or pharynx or anaphylaxis.

87. How does the future look for asthma immunotherapy?

Research is continuing on new approaches to developing immunomodulators for asthma that target regulator molecules that affect inflammation.

However, there are two major limitations on the use of immunomodulators. First, immunotherapies are expensive, and health services can have difficulty in funding these therapies. Second, asthma is a very diverse and varied disease, so it is necessary to determine which asthma types will benefit from a particular therapy with immunomodulators. The focused nature of immunotherapies limits their broad application.

88. When should long-acting beta$_2$-agonists be used?

Beta$_2$-agonists act on smooth muscle cells in the airways causing muscle relaxation and, through that, bronchodilation. Two general types of beta$_2$-agonists are in use—short term and long term. Short-acting beta$_2$-agonists (SABAs), as the name implies, have a rapid onset of action, and are used for quick relief of symptoms due to bronchoconstriction. SABAs will be discussed in Question 90.

Long-acting beta$_2$-agonists (LABAs) have a more prolonged duration of action than SABAs, lasting at least 12 hours. LABAs are designed to prevent symptoms. Currently, two LABA medications are widely available, salmeterol and eformoterol. Both medications have similar clinical effects when used regularly. Salmeterol has a slower onset of action, less total bronchodilator action at high dose, and less likelihood of tachyphylaxis (rapidly decreasing response to the medication). Eformoterol, on the other hand, has a faster onset of action, greater bronchodilator action at high dose, and a greater likelihood of tachyphylaxis. Both LABAs tend to develop tachyphylaxis when used on a regular basis. Although LABAs have a bronchodilator action, they also have an anti-inflammatory effect when used in combination with ICSs.

EPR-3 recommends that LABAs be used in the following manner:
- LABAs should not be used as the only therapy for long-term control of asthma.
- LABAs can be used in combination with ICSs for long-term control and prevention of symptoms in moderate or severe persistent asthma in children ≥5 years of age and adults.
- Compared to other medications available, LABA is the preferred medication to combine with ICS in youths ≥12 years of age and adults.

- The beneficial effects of LABA in combination therapy for patients who require more therapy than low-dose ICS alone to control asthma should be weighed against the increased risk of severe exacerbations, although uncommon, associated with the daily use of LABAs.

    – For patients ≥5 years of age who have moderate persistent asthma or asthma inadequately controlled on low-dose ICS, the option to increase the ICS dose should be given equal weight to the option of adding LABA.

    – For patients ≥5 years of age who have severe persistent asthma or asthma inadequately controlled, the combination of LABA and ICS is the preferred therapy.
- LABA may be used before exercise to prevent exercise-induced bronchospasm (EIB), but the duration of action does not exceed 5 hours with chronic regular use. Frequent and chronic use of LABA for EIB is discouraged because this use may disguise poorly controlled persistent asthma.
- The use of LABA for the treatment of acute symptoms or exacerbations is not currently recommended.

Extensive Cochrane systematic reviews on the use of LABAs led to the following conclusions on the use of LABAs:
- LABAs are effective and safe when regularly used in patients with chronic asthma.
- Regular use of LABAs did not result in any lessening of asthma control; in fact, there was a lessening of exacerbation rates.
- Studies support the use of LABAs in addition to ICSs as recommended in current guidelines.
- The use of LABAs without ICSs may have beneficial effects without increasing the risk of side effects.
- Regular use of LABAs have advantages over SABAs regarding clinical outcomes.
- Under some situations, long-term use of high doses of ICSs can result in increased absorption of the medicine into the systemic circulation with accompanying adverse side effects. When LABAs are used with ICSs, the doses of ICSs needed to control asthma may be reduced, lessening the possibility of adverse side effects.

89. What are methylxanthines?

Methylxanthines are a chemical class of drugs related to the caffeine family. Oral theophylline is the principally used methylxanthine. Theophylline provides mild to moderate bronchodilation (depending on dose) in persons who have asthma. Theophylline exhibits mild anti-inflammatory activity and a small effect on airway reactivity. Theophylline has found use as a supplemental therapy to ICS, particularly with issues related to cost or a patient's aversion to inhaled medication.

Theophylline is most effective in controlling asthma symptoms if a steady blood level can be maintained. Sustained-release capsules or tablets that release medication over many hours are an effective way to administer the medication. This method of administration is particularly useful in controlling nighttime asthma.

Theophylline is notable for causing a variety of adverse side effects. The dosage of theophylline is critical, as there is a narrow range between the dosage required to alleviate symptoms and the level that can cause toxic symptoms. During treatment, it is essential to monitor the serum concentrations of theophylline to ensure that toxic concentrations are avoided. Individual patients can vary in their response to theophylline, such as health status and environmental influences. Other medications can change the way the body metabolizes theophylline, which could lead to toxic levels of the medication.

Your physician will ask the following questions before prescribing theophylline:
- What prescription medications are you are taking?
- What nonprescription medications and vitamins are you are taking, including ephedrine, epinephrine, phenylephrine, phenylpropanolamine, or pseudoephedrine? Many nonprescription products contain these drugs (e.g., diet pills and medications for colds and asthma), so check labels carefully. Do not take these medications without talking to your doctor; they can increase the side effects of theophylline.
- Do you have or have ever had seizures, ulcers, heart disease, an overactive or underactive thyroid gland, high

blood pressure, or liver disease or do you have a history of alcohol abuse?

- Are you pregnant, plan to become pregnant, or are breast-feeding? If you become pregnant while taking theophylline, call your doctor.
- Do you use tobacco products? Cigarette smoking may decrease the effectiveness of theophylline.

Talk to your doctor if the following symptoms are severe or do not go away:

- Upset stomach
- Stomach pain
- Diarrhea
- Headache
- Restlessness
- Insomnia
- Irritability

Call your doctor immediately if you experience any of the following symptoms:

- Vomiting
- Increased or rapid heart rate
- Irregular heartbeat
- Seizures
- Skin rash

90. What are the quick-relief medications?

a. Short-acting beta$_2$-agonists (SABAs) are the drug of choice for treating acute asthma symptoms and exacerbations and for preventing exercise-induced bronchospasm or nocturnal asthma. Beta agonists reverse the tightness or constriction in the bronchial tubes. They do not reduce inflammation. SABAs are short for beta-adrenergic agonists, so-named because they activate the beta-2 receptors located on the bronchial smooth muscle inducing relaxation. Beta-adrenoreceptor agonists mimic the action of epinephrine and norepinephrine signaling in the heart, lungs, and smooth muscle tissue, with epinephrine expressing the highest affinity. SABAs cause a prompt (within 3–5 minutes) increase in airflow. As you will recall, the frequency of beta-agonist use is an important criterion in classifying asthma severity and control in asthma patients.

Increasing use of SABA treatment or using SABA >2 days a week for symptom relief (not prevention of EIB) indicates inadequate control of asthma and the need for initiating or intensifying anti-inflammatory therapy. Using SABA on a regular basis can lead to decreased responsiveness of the medication (tachyphylaxis) due to desensitization of the beta$_2$ receptors in the lungs.

Table 11.7 Characteristics of short-acting beta$_2$-agonists

Generic Name	Trade Name	Administration	Clinical Issues
Albuterol sulfate	Proventil HFA Ventolin HFA ProAir HFA	Metered-dose Inhaler Solution for nebulization Oral solution	Most commonly used bronchodilator commonly used in rescue therapy for exacerbations. Prolonged use may be associated with tachyphylaxis
Levabuterol (related chemically to albuterol sulfate)	Xopenex	(Same as albuterol sulfate)	Effective in smaller doses than albuterol The dose may be doubled in acute severe episodes when even a slight increase in the bronchodilator response may make a big difference in the management strategy
Pirbuterol	Maxair Autoinhaler	Metered-dose inhaler Breath-actuated inhaler	The ease of administration with the breath-actuated device makes it an attractive choice in the treatment of acute symptoms in younger children, who otherwise may not be able to use a metered-dose inhaler

Use of beta$_2$-agonists can result in mild to moderate adverse effects, including the following:
- Anxiety
- Tremor (your hand or another part of your body may shake)
- Restlessness
- Headache

- Fast and irregular heartbeats. Call your doctor right away if you have this side effect.
  b. Should the asthma patient be cautious about using beta blockers?

Beta blockers are widely prescribed for the management of cardiovascular disease. Beta blockers are used for acute coronary syndrome, to prevent secondary coronary events, as well as for management of angina and cardiac arrhythmias. Beta blockers have also found use in the management of anxiety, migraine, and preeclampsia.

Some patients with asthma may also have heart or other conditions that could be treated with beta blockers. For many decades, physicians were reluctant to prescribe beta blockers to these patients as they felt it would block the beta2 receptor in the bronchial smooth muscle, thereby counteracting the action of SABAs, and possibly triggering exacerbations.

Continuing research has led to a better understanding of the action of beta blockers and to more selective and effective products. There are two types of beta blockers, $beta_1$ and $beta_2$. $Beta_1$ receptors dominate in the heart, while $beta_2$ receptors dominate in the bronchial smooth muscle. The early beta blockers were "nonselective," meaning that they blocked the activity of both $beta_1$ and $beta_2$ receptors, thereby affecting other organs such as the lungs in addition to the heart. Cardioselective beta blockers, or $beta_1$ blockers, have more than 20 times more affinity for $beta_1$ receptors than for $beta_2$ receptors, whereas nonselective beta blockers have equal affinity for both receptors. Many studies and clinical experience have shown that cardioselective $beta_1$ blockers can be safely given to asthma patients with little or no adverse effects, as they have minimal effect in blocking beta2 receptors in bronchial smooth muscle.

Beta blockers act by interfering with epinephrine (adrenaline), a hormone that normally stimulates the heart to beat faster and stronger. Beta blockers slow the heart rate and decrease cardiac output, lowering blood pressure and decreasing the amount of work the heart must do. By lowering the oxygen needs of the heart, beta blockers help prevent or relieve ischemia (deficiency in the supply of blood to the heart muscle).

Table 11.8 Cardioselective beta$_1$ blockers

Generic Name	Trade Name
betaxolol	Kerlone
acebutol	Sectral
atenolol	Tenormin
metoprolol	Toprol-XL Lopressor Metoprolol Succinate ER Metoprolol Tartrate
bisprolol	Zebeta
nebivolol	Bystolic
esmolol	Brevibloc

Beta blockers act in a manner opposite to that of beta agonists. Beta agonists stimulate receptors in bronchial smooth muscle leading to bronchodilation and protection against release of bronchoconstrictors.

c. Anticholinergic drugs act by blocking the release of acetylcholine from cholinergic receptors located on parasympathetic nerves (vagus nerves) in the airways (see Question 4). The asthmatic condition results in dysfunctional receptors leading to an excessive release of acetylcholine. The increased supply of acetylcholine activates receptors located on bronchial smooth muscle, submucosal glands, and blood vessels to cause bronchoconstriction, mucus secretion, and vasodilation.

Anticholinergic medicines block the activity of the parasympathetic nerve receptors, resulting in relaxation of the bronchial smooth muscle.

Cholinergic means stimulated, activated, or transmitted by acetylcholine. In asthma, the term applies to parasympathetic nerve fibers that release acetylcholine when a nerve impulse passes.

Anticholinergic medications are more commonly used to treat bronchoconstriction in COPD patients and have received FDA approval for this use. Physicians may use anticholinergics for asthma patients by "off-label" use, a common practice. The use of anticholinergics to treat asthma is relatively recent and may be considered as a supplementary treatment for asthma patients whose asthma is poorly controlled.

The first anticholinergic medication to be introduced was ipratropium bromide, for short-acting use. Most studies have shown that ipratropium bromide is less effective than beta$_2$-agonists in relieving asthmatic symptoms. These results have led to the opinion that asthma medications that treat inflammation (beta$_2$-agonists) are more effective than medications that reduce smooth muscle tone (anticholinergics).

EPR-3 concluded that ipratropium bromide, administered in multiple doses along with SABA in moderate or severe asthma exacerbations in the ED, provides additive benefit. Patients who have more severe obstruction of airways appear to benefit the most. Ipratropium bromide has been used, with some success, as a quick-relief medication to avoid the use of as-needed albuterol in clinical research trials in patients who have mild asthma.

Tiotropium bromide is the first long-acting inhaled anticholinergic drug that was developed in the 1990s and is approved for the long-term management of stable COPD. Some studies have shown potential with this drug for the treatment of asthma.

   d. Systemic corticosteroids

      As discussed in Question 84, the long-term use of systemic corticosteroids can lead to a large variety of adverse side effects. Using systemic corticosteroids on a short-term basis (less than 2 weeks) largely avoids these problems.

Systemic corticosteroids have a place as short-acting medications for moderate or severe exacerbations to prevent progression of exacerbation, reverse inflammation, speed recovery, and reduce the rate of relapse. To be fully effective, the medication should be given as soon as possible after arriving in the emergency department. Short-term therapy should continue until patient's symptoms resolve, usually requiring 3–10 days but may require longer.

Apparently, oral corticosteroids are not very effective for young children, ages 0–5; however, the medicines may be helpful in gaining rapid asthma control in older children. Oral corticosteroid use in adults for 5–10 days is effective in regaining control of asthma after acute flare-ups.

Systemic corticosteroids are usually given orally (as pills or liquid).The medications may be given intravenously or intramuscularly in emergency departments to manage acute asthma. Some studies have shown that giving prednisolone orally is as effective as giving the medication by injection. The most commonly used systemic corticosteroids used on a short-term basis are as follows:

Generic Name	Brand Name
methylprednisolone	Medrol Medrol Dosepak
prednisolone	Pediapred Prelone
prednisone	Rayos Sterapred

The three drugs have similar chemical compositions and closely resemble natural cortisol. Prednisolone and prednisone are more commonly used than methylprednisolone.

91. Should I use complementary or alternative medicine to treat my asthma?

Complementary and alternative medicine use approaches to treatment that were developed outside of mainstream Western, or conventional, medicine. Complementary medicine practices are used together with conventional medicine, while alternative medicine practices are used in place of conventional medicine. The medical establishment does not recommend the replacement of standard therapies with alternative medicine.

Studies have shown that a large percentage of asthma patients use complementary medicine, but that they still adhere to conventional asthma treatment use. It is important for patients to discuss with their doctor regarding complementary medicine use.

EPR-3 does not recommend the use of acupuncture, chiropractic therapy, yoga, or homeopathy for the treatment of asthma.

EPR-3 concluded that there is insufficient evidence to recommend herbal and other natural products for treating asthma. Since herbal products are not standardized, one must be aware that some may have harmful ingredients and that some may interact with other pharmaceutical products that the patient may be taking. Some natural products may enhance the effect of standard products to the point that they are toxic. Using some natural products may result in patients not using more effective standard products.

ASHMI is an extract of three Chinese herbs that has shown promise in improving lung function and in reducing clinical symptoms of asthma in some studies. ASHMI has received approval as an FDA Investigational New Drug and is now undergoing clinical studies. Ding Chuan Tang is another Chinese herbal preparation that has shown promise in reducing airway hyperresponsiveness.

Although the use of natural products for treating asthma has not been thoroughly evaluated, some individual patients may benefit. The following are a few products that have been used:
- Garlic has anti-inflammatory properties.
- Ginger also has anti-inflammatory properties, and has shown in a recent study to result in a reduction of asthma symptoms. The study didn't show, however, that ginger use led to any improvement in actual lung function.
- Tumeric has been found to have some anti-allergy properties. Tumeric may have an effect on histamines.
- Omega-3 fatty acids may help to decrease airway inflammation and boost lung function, according to some studies.
- Echinacea and licorice root are not recommended due to the risk of side effects.

EPR-3 concluded that some studies suggest that breathing exercises may provide benefits in reducing SABA use, quality of use, and in number of exacerbations.

Preliminary data suggest that relaxation techniques may help improve not only symptoms (which in studies appeared to improve nonspecifically) but also lung function.

 ON THE WEB

For an article on "A Systematic Review of Complementary and Alternative Medicine for Asthma Self-Management," please visit:
https://www.ncbi.nlm.nih.gov/pmc/articles/PMC3859131/

92. What are the prospects for new asthma medicines?

Although highly effective asthma therapies are currently available, over half of patients with asthma appear to be poorly controlled. A major problem in this regard is that patients prefer oral medication over inhaled medications, even though the risk of side effects is greater by using the oral route. When patients take ICSs with or without long-acting beta$_2$-agonists according to schedule, their asthma is well controlled.

Leading researchers in academia and the pharmaceutical industry have determined that new drugs are needed for asthma to include: new classes of drugs that are effective in severe, poorly controlled asthma; an oral treatment that is as effective as ICSs but without any side effects; and drugs that modify the course or even cure the disease.

The following are current approaches to new drug development:
- New long-acting beta$_2$-agonists-bronchodilators are important for preventing and relieving bronchoconstriction but have been notable for their short duration of action. The introduction of the LABAs salmeterol and formoterol which last over 12 hours was considered to be a major advance. Three even longer-acting beta$_2$-agonists, indacaterol, vilanterol, and olodaterol, have been approved for use in COPD. These "ultra-LABAs" have duration of action of 24 hours or more and are suitable for once-daily dosing.
- New corticosteroids—Although ICSs are the most effective anti-inflammatory medicines for asthma, concern remains for the potential for systemic side effects from their use. Since most of the adverse side effects are due to the hormonal effects of steroids, research has been directed toward developing molecules known as dissociated steroids that attempt to separate the side-effect mechanisms from the anti-inflammatory mechanisms. However, new medications based on this principle have yet to reach the market.
- Specific immunotherapy—Treatment of allergy by subcutaneous injection of allergen is not very effective in controlling asthma and could lead to anaphylactic shock. Developing medications that modify and suppress the

immunologic process are possibilities.

- Targeting mediators of inflammation—The complex inflammatory processes in asthma involve a wide variety of chemical mediators that can be targeted and inactivated by drugs. These new drugs under development are nonsteroidal in action and could be particularly effective for patients with severe asthma who are poorly responsive to corticosteroids.
- Cytokines as therapy—Interestingly, some cytokines, such as interleukins and interferons, are inhibitory to the inflammatory process, and whose secretion may be defective in some patients. Providing these cytokines in inhaled medications may be a possibility.

Medications for comorbid conditions

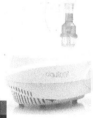

Comorbid conditions are medical conditions that occur together with asthma. These conditions can make asthma worse, and under some circumstances, may even provoke asthma. It is very important, therefore, to treat comorbid conditions.

93. How can I treat allergic rhinitis?

As mentioned in Question 26, allergic rhinitis (commonly known as hay fever) is an inflammation of the nasal mucus membranes.

Allergic rhinitis can be treated by the following methods:
- Antihistamines are the primary means to control rhinitis. Antihistamines reduce or block histamines that are released as part of the allergic reaction (Question 28). Antihistamines treat the symptoms of allergic reactions. Older antihistamines (called first generation) were sedating, while newer second-generation antihistamines are non-sedating or less sedating but may still cause drowsiness in some people. Antihistamines come in many forms, including tablets, capsules, nasal sprays, and eyedrops. A very large number of antihistamines are available, either over the counter or by prescription.
- Decongestants are medications used to relieve stuffy noses. They are available in either oral form (tablets,

capsules, or liquids), or as nasal sprays or nose drops. Nasal sprays should only be used occasionally, as prolonged use can irritate and inflame the nasal passages making congestion worse. The active ingredient in most decongestants is either pseudoephedrine or phenylephrine. Antihistamines and decongestants are often combined in one medication.

- Cromolyn sodium acts by stabilizing mast cells preventing the release of histamine and other inflammatory mediators. Cromolyn sodium is available over the counter as a nasal spray or powder. The medication is most useful to allergy sufferers if used beginning 2 to 4 weeks before exposure to allergens. The medication can be used to treat seasonal as well as chronic allergic rhinitis. Allergy specialists like cromolyn sulfate as an alternative treatment due to its excellent safety record: it is well tolerated, is poorly absorbed systematically, and is not associated with drug interactions.

94. How can I treat sinusitis?

As discussed in Question 23, the sinuses are hollow cavities in the bones that surround your nasal cavity. Sinusitis is an inflammation of the sinuses that can be due to viruses, bacteria, or fungi.

Sinusitis can be caused by:
- Upper respiratory tract viral infections such as the common cold. These infections are the most frequent causes of sinusitis.
- Bacteria.
- Fungal infections in patients on long-term antibiotic treatment or who have been taking oral corticosteroids on a chronic basis.

The main symptoms of sinusitis include pain and pressure in the face along with a stuffy or a runny nose. Other symptoms include headache, fever, yellowish or greenish discharge from the nose, cough that produces mucus, and tooth pain.

Sinusitis can be acute, lasting for around 3–4 weeks, or chronic, which can last for months.

Treatment of sinusitis depends on the type of infection. Antibiotics are only useful for bacterial infections, while antifungal medications can be helpful for fungal infections.

Home remedies for sinusitis may very well be recommended by your physician. You should keep in mind that these remedies work just to relieve symptoms, not to cure sinusitis.

These remedies include:
- Irrigation of your nostrils with warm saline water. Various nasal wash devices are available in your neighborhood pharmacy.
- Steam inhalation to liquefy and soften crusty mucus while moisturizing inflamed passages.

95. Will treatment of GERD alleviate asthma symptoms?

A large percentage of asthma patients also experience GERD symptoms. In Question 21, we described how GERD could affect asthma through aspiration of microdroplets of acid reflux into the lungs.

Asthma, in turn, can also worsen GERD symptoms. The most common theory is that pressure swings in the thorax of asthmatics allow more acid to reflux into the esophagus. Some asthma medications can increase heartburn and other symptoms of GERD. Theophylline has been most closely tied to worsening GERD symptoms. Bronchodilators may reduce the lower esophageal sphincter pressure and trigger GERD symptoms.

If you are experiencing symptoms of GERD, be sure to tell your doctor. He or she can investigate the possibility that GERD is contributing to your asthma symptoms. Treatment of GERD symptoms has found to result in improved quality of life for asthma patients, and possibly a reduced frequency of exacerbations.

Patients with symptoms of GERD (heartburn) usually begin by taking antacids, but this measure is usually only partially effective. When GERD becomes more severe and chronic, patients can take more effective GERD medications. H2 blockers are available over the counter and by prescription and are known by such trade names as Tagamet, Zantac, Axid, and Pepsid. The newer proton pump inhibitors are considered more effective and are known by such trade names as Prilosec, Zegerid, and Prevacid.

There are many steps patients can take to alleviate GERD, such as:

- Avoid eating heavy meals within 3 hours before going to bed. This measure is to assure you do not go to bed on a full stomach.
- Reduce consumption of foods and beverages that are thought to aggravate GERD. These include chocolate, peppermint, alcohol, coffee, tea, and carbonated beverages.
- Avoid smoking.
- Sleep on your bed with head elevated, preferably by raising the bed with blocks. Adding pillows under your head is less effective. The purpose of this procedure is to keep your stomach contents below the point where you could inhale them while sleeping.

REFERENCES

References

CHAPTER 8

1. National Asthma Education and Prevention Program. "Expert Panel Report 3: Guidelines for the Diagnosis and Management of Asthma." National Heart, Lung, and Blood Institute. (2007). *http://www.nhlbi.nih.gov/files/docs/guidelines/asthgdln.pdf.*

CHAPTER 9

2. Pollart, Susan and Elward Kurtis. "Overview of changes to asthma guidelines: diagnosis and treatment." *Am Family Physician.* 79, no. 9 (2009): 761–767. *http://www.aafp.org/afp/2009/0501/p761.pdf*

CHAPTER 10

3. National Asthma Education and Prevention Program. "Expert Panel Report 3: Guidelines for the Diagnosis and Management of Asthma." National Heart, Lung, and Blood Institute. (2007). *http://www.nhlbi.nih.gov/files/docs/guidelines/asthgdln.pdf*

CHAPTER 11

4. Arunthari, Vichaya, Bruinsma R, Lee A, and Johnson M. "A prospective, comparative trial of standard and breath-actuated nebulizer: efficacy, safety, and satisfaction." *Respiratory Care.* 57, no. 8 (2012):1242-1247.

https://www.ncbi.nlm.nih.gov/pubmed/22348319

5. Barnes, Peter. "TH2 cytokines and asthma: an introduction." *Respir Res.* 2 (2001):64–65.
    https://www.ncbi.nlm.nih.gov/pmc/articles/PMC59569/

6. Clark T, Godfrey S, Lee T, Thomson N. *Asthma.* Arnold Publishers. (2000).
    www.arnoldpublishers.com

7. National Education and Prevention Program. "Asthma tipsheets." National Heart, Lung, and Blood Institute. March 2013.
    https://www.nhlbi.nih.gov/files/docs/public/lung/asthma_tipsheets. pdf

8. Hossny, Elham, Nelson Rosario, Bee Wah Lee, Meenu Singh, Dalia El-Ghoneimy, Jian Yi SOH and Peter Le Souef. "The use of inhaled corticosteroids in pediatric asthma: update." *World Allergy Organization Journal.* 9, no.26 (2016):1–24.
    https://waojournal.biomedcentral.com/articles/10.1186/s40413-016-0117-0

9. Li, Xiu-Min. "Treatment of asthma and food allergy with herbal interventions from traditional Chinese medicine." *Mt Sinai J Med.* 78, no.5 (2011):697-716.
    https://www.ncbi.nlm.nih.gov/pmc/articles/PMC4118473/

10. Philip, Julie, Judy Maselli, Lee Pachter, and Michael Cabana. "Complementary and alternative medicine use and adherence with pediatric asthma treatment." *Pediatrics.* 129, no. 5 (2012):1148–1154.
    https://www.ncbi.nlm.nih.gov/pmc/articles/PMC4074611/pdf/ peds.2011-2467.pdf

11. Reddy, Sumathi. "Many asthma patients use their inhalers incorrectly, research shows." *The Wall Street Journal. March 6, 2017.*
    https://www.wsj.com/articles/many-asthma-patients-use-their-inhalers-incorrectly-research-shows-1488822193

12. Walters, J, Wood-Baker, and Walters, E. "Long-acting beta2-agonists in asthma: an overview of Cochrane systematic reviews." *Respiratory Medicine.* 99 (2005):384-395.
    https://www.ncbi.nlm.nih.gov/pubmed/?term=Long-acting+beta2-agoni sts+in+asthma%3A+an+overview+of+Cochrane+systematic+reviews.

CHAPTER 12

13. Mastronarde, John. "Is there a relationship between GERD and asthma?" *Gastroenterology & Hepatology.* 8, no. 6 (2012):401–403.
    https://www.ncbi.nlm.nih.gov/pmc/articles/PMC3424477/pdf/GH-08-401.pdf

14. Ratner, P. Ehrlich P, Fineman S, Meltzer E, and Skoner DP. "Use of intranasal cromolyn sodium for allergic rhinitis." *Mayo Clinic Proc.* 77, no. 4 (2002):350–354.
    https://www.ncbi.nlm.nih.gov/pubmed/11936930

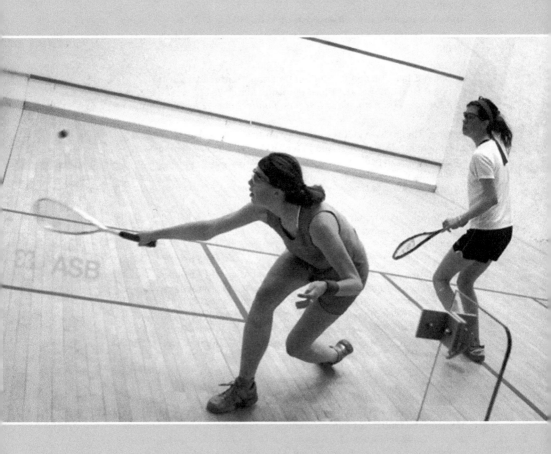

PART FIVE

Asthma Management and Lifestyle

In Part Five, we discuss the *Education for a Partnership in Asthma Care* program, the Asthma Action Plan, a healthy lifestyle, special concerns of the asthma patient during childhood and pregnancy, and traveling with asthma.

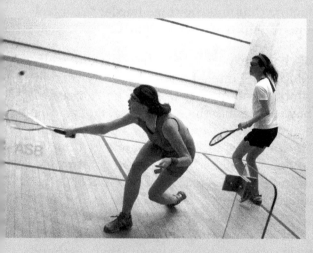

Credit: Steve McFarland
Creative Commons

Education for a partnership in asthma care

96. What is the importance of patient education in asthma care?

Education for a Partnership in Asthma Care requires education for the patient or caregiver about asthma self-management. The program also requires education for clinicians to enhance their skills in teaching patients self-management and provide support to implement guidelines-recommended practices. Recommendations are presented on asthma self-management, education at multiple points of care, tools for asthma self-management, and provider education.

Evidence is now abundant that asthma self-management education is effective in improving outcomes of chronic asthma. Specific training in self-management skills is necessary to produce behavior that modifies the outcomes of chronic illnesses such as asthma. Expert care, with regular review by health professionals, is necessary but not sufficient to improve outcomes. Patients must actively participate in their own care, which means consciously using strategies and taking actions to minimize exposure to factors that make asthma harder to control and adjusting treatments to improve disease control.

The ultimate goal of both expert care and patient self-management is to reduce the impact of asthma on related morbidity, functional ability, and quality of life. The benefits of educating people who have asthma in the self-management skills of self-assessment, use of medications, and actions to prevent or control exacerbations include a reduction in urgent care visits and hospitalizations, reduction of asthma-related health care costs, and improvement in health status. Other benefits of value from self-management education are a reduction in symptoms, less limitation of activity, improvement in the quality of life and perceived control of asthma, and improved medication adherence. Cost-analysis studies have shown that asthma education can be delivered in a cost-effective manner and that morbidity is reduced as a result, especially in high-risk subjects.

Although not all controlled trials of asthma self-management education have shown positive results, it is notable that controlled studies have demonstrated benefit from patient education programs delivered in a wide range of points of care, including clinics, EDs, hospitals, pharmacies, doctors' offices, schools, and community settings. These results have been achieved through face-to-face educational strategies and the use of new electronic technologies. Referenced studies are from multiple countries. Some outcomes may be dependent on the context of care and may not be completely generalizable.

97. Are written asthma action plans useful?

The previous question summarized the importance of patient education in managing their asthma. EPR-3 formalized the process by recommending the use of a written Asthma Action Plan.

The National Heart, Lung, and Blood Institute prepared a sample Asthma Action Plan. Please visit: https://www.nhlbi.nih.gov/files/docs/public/lung/asthma_actplan.pdf

The NHLBI Asthma Action Plan is designed to be a concise set of instructions for a patient to follow for self-management of his or her asthma. The Plan is divided into three conditions of a patient's asthma progressing from a stable condition to a medical emergency. Within each condition, instructions are provided on medications and other actions to take.

Although the NHLBI Asthma Action Plan is a good starting point, both physicians and patients agree that a more personalized action plan should be drawn up that reflects the unique features of the patient's asthma. The written action plan must emphasize two features: (1) daily management, and (2) how to recognize and handle worsening asthma, including self-adjustment of medications in response to acute symptoms or changes in PEF measures. Written asthma action plans are particularly recommended for patients who have moderate or severe persistent asthma, a history of severe exacerbations, or poorly controlled asthma. Any action plan drawn up should be a result of collaboration between the doctor and patient.

The action plan should be a dynamic document, reviewed and modified according to the changing conditions of the patient's asthma.

The action plan should represent only part of the partnership between doctor and patient. Specific training in self-management skills is necessary to produce behavior that modifies the outcomes of chronic illnesses such as asthma. Studies have shown no significant differences in hospitalizations, ED visits, unscheduled doctor's visits, or frequency of nocturnal asthma symptoms among patients who self-adjusted their medication to patients whose medications were adjusted by their physicians. The benefits of educating people who have asthma in the self-management skills of self-assessment, use of medications, and actions to prevent or control exacerbations include reduction in urgent care visits and hospitalizations, reduction of asthma-related health care costs, and improvement in health status.

Studies have shown that self-management education for the patient that included a written asthma action plan appeared more effective than other forms of self-management education.

In addition to the primary physician, other medical professionals can become involved in patient self-management education. These professionals can include specially trained nurses, emergency department personnel, and respiratory therapists.

CHAPTER 14 *Occupational asthma*

98. What is occupational asthma?

Occupational asthma is due to exposure to many types of chemicals and dust in the workplace environment. The resultant asthma may be a new onset of asthma due to exposure to certain substances found in the workplace or an aggravation of a preexisting condition. Many of these substances are uniquely found in the workplace. Up to 15% of asthma cases in the U.S. may be work-related.

99. What workers are at risk for workplace asthma?

Substances that directly irritate the airways can include chemicals, fumes, gasses, aerosols, paints, and smoke. The Occupational Safety and Health Administration (OSHA) has determined that a group of chemicals called isocyanates are one of the most common chemical causes of work-related asthma.

Many occupations involve exposure to biologic materials such as wood products, textiles, and food products that contain allergens that can trigger allergic responses. Allergy to latex gloves is becoming increasingly important.

The following workers are at higher risk:
- Bakers
- Detergent manufacturers
- Drug manufacturers
- Farmers
- Grain elevator workers
- Laboratory workers (especially those working with laboratory animals)
- Metal workers
- Millers
- Plastics workers
- Woodworkers

 ON THE WEB Wikipedia provides an extensive list of occupations and main substances involved in provoking occupational asthma. Visit: https://en.wikipedia.org/wiki/Occupational_asthma

100. How does a physician determine if a patient's symptoms are work-related?

The physician will ask the patient questions about the work environment, as well as try to relate the patient's symptoms to his or her work exposure.

Potential for workplace-related symptoms:
- Materials are present in the workplace that are known to provoke asthma (e.g., isocyanates, plant or animal products).
- Irritants or physical stimuli are present (e.g., cold/heat, dust, humidity).
- Co-workers may have similar symptoms.

Patterns of symptoms (about work exposures):
- Symptoms started when you changed jobs.
- Chemicals and other conditions at your workplace make it difficult to breathe.
- Improvement occurs during vacations or days off (may take a week or more).

- Symptoms occur shortly after you are exposed to the substance. The symptoms often improve or go away when you leave work.
- Symptoms may be immediate (<1 hour), delayed (most commonly, 2–8 hours after exposure), or nocturnal.
- Initial symptoms may occur after high-level exposure (e.g., spill).

If the patient already has a diagnosis of asthma, the physician may request the patient to record data to determine if airflow limitation is work-related. The physician may further order certain diagnostic tests as follows.
- Record data for 2–3 weeks (2 weeks at work and up to 1 week off work, as needed to identify or exclude work-related changes in PEF):
  - Record when symptoms and exposures occur.
  - Record when a bronchodilator is used.
  - Measure and record peak flow (or FEV1) every 2 hours while awake.
- Immunologic (allergic) tests.
- Spirometry tests to help confirm diagnosis and track lung function over time.
- Specific inhalation challenge tests to identify the occupational origin of asthma. The tests involve breathing in small quantities of industrial agents that may induce an exacerbation. The test is safe when performed by physicians with appropriate expertise.

101. How do you treat occupational asthma?

Work-aggravated asthma:
- Work with onsite health care providers or managers/supervisors.
- Discuss avoidance, ventilation, respiratory protection, smoke-free tobacco environment.

Occupationally induced asthma:
- Recommend complete cessation of exposure to initiating agent. Occupational asthma may keep getting worse if you continue to be exposed to the substance that is causing the problem, even if medicines improve your symptoms.
- Move to a different location at the work site where there is less exposure to the substance. Moving may help, but

over time, even a very small amount of the substance can trigger an asthma attack.

- Using a respiratory device to protect or reduce your exposure may help.
- Changing your job may be the last recourse if the asthma persists.

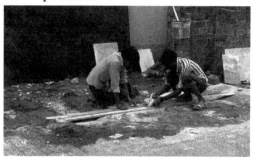

▲ **Figure 14.1**
Stonecutters working without protective face mask
Credit: Abhishek 727
Creative Commons

Taking measures to protect against dust, chemicals, and other irritants present in the workplace are very important for the asthma sufferer.

Special considerations for the athlete who has asthma

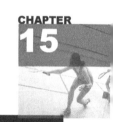

102. What sports more likely to provoke exercise-induced bronchoconstriction (EIB) in the athlete?

As discussed in Question 46, the asthma patient is more likely to experience bronchoconstriction after strong, vigorous exercise. Many people with chronic asthma will have already experienced severe breathing problems after doing sports. But sometimes people who do not have asthma also have these kinds of symptoms after doing sports.

NOTE

The asthma patient should be encouraged to participate in exercise and sports activities. It is just as important to take the necessary precautions and preparations.

When we breathe in, our nose cleans, warms, and moistens the air. During physical exercise, though, we breathe faster, deeper, and more through our mouth. As a result, the air that enters our lungs is colder and drier than usual. The membranes lining the bronchi (lung airway passages) might swell up as a result. In people with asthma, these membranes are already very sensitive, and they tend to react very strongly. Cold and dry air can heighten this effect.

Few studies have been done to determine which sports are more likely to trigger EIB. Our discussion on the effect of cold, dry air would indicate that athletes that engage in outdoor sports such as skiing or ice hockey would be more subject to EIB. Athletes engaged in swimming where the air is warm and moist may be less likely to experience EIB.

Inhalers and emergency medications should always be available during exercise and sports activities for the student with asthma.

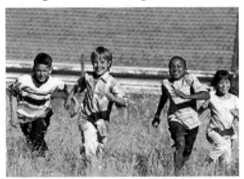

▲ **Figure 15.1**
Exercise is important for all children
Source: CDCCopyright: Lopolo/Shutterstock

103. What medications are best to prevent or control EIB?

If your asthma medication has been adapted to your specific situation and you can effectively control your asthma, you are far less likely to have sudden breathing difficulties when you do sports. Your doctor can help you find the medication that best suits your physical activities.

There are two main groups of asthma medications: controllers and relievers. Controller or "preventer" medication is used as a long-term treatment to "control" asthma. The effect of this medication is felt slowly over time. Reliever or "rescue" medication has a short-term effect. The medication can be used before doing strenuous physical activities, as well as to relieve acute asthma attacks. For safety reasons, though, it is important to talk to your doctor about how often you can use reliever medication on one day.

The following medications can be used before strenuous activities to prevent EIB:

- Short-acting beta$_2$-agonists are inhaled as a spray and have a fast effect. They cause the airways to expand, making it easier to breathe. When used just before strenuous physical activities, they can prevent an asthma attack. The effect is strongest about 30 minutes after being inhaled and lasts about 3 to 5 hours. Short-acting beta$_2$-agonists can also be used to treat exacerbations: They start working after a few minutes and can help you breathe better.
- Leukotriene antagonists: These medications, taken in the form of tablets, block the effect of leukotrienes. Leukotrienes are chemical messengers that play a key role in the inflammatory response in the airways. They can be used before strenuous activities to prevent exercise-induced asthma.
- Mast cell stabilizers (cromones) are inhaled using a puffer. They reduce allergic and inflammatory reactions by preventing the release of histamine from the body's cells. Histamine is a chemical messenger that also plays a key role in allergic reactions. But cromones are not as good at preventing exercise-induced asthma as beta$_2$-agonists are. Even when used together with short-acting beta$_2$-agonists, they do not work better than beta$_2$-agonists alone.
- Anticholinergics affect the nervous system, causing the bronchi to dilate (open up). They can help in exercise-induced asthma, too. But they are not as good at preventing exercise-related breathing problems as beta$_2$-agonists and mast cell stabilizers are.

It is often not easy to find out which medications best prevent exercise-induced asthma in a person. You may have to try out different medications to find out which medication is right for you.

CHAPTER 16

Controlling environmental factors that make asthma worse

104. What is meant by environmental factors?

In this chapter, environmental factors refer to allergens, pollutants, and irritants present in the home or outdoors. Work-related factors were discussed in Chapter 11.

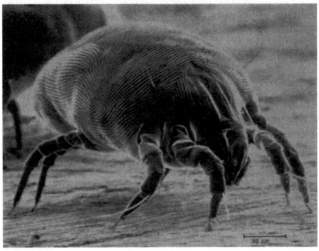

▲ **Figure 16.1**
House dust mite
Credit: FDA/Creative Commons

House-dust mites are universal in areas of high humidity (most areas of the United States) but are usually not present at high altitudes or in arid areas unless moisture is added to the indoor air.

105. What measures can you take to control environmental factors that can make asthma worse?

Allergens

Reduce or eliminate exposure to the allergen the patient is sensitive to, including:
- Pet allergens: All warm-blooded pets, such as cats, dogs, birds, and rodents, have dead skin cells (animal dander)

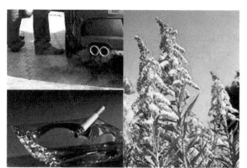

◀ Figure 16.2
Common asthma triggers

Centers for Disease Control and Prevention
https://www.cdc.gov/asthma/triggers.html

and make urine or stool. All of these animal materials can contain allergens and trigger asthma symptoms. The following steps can help to reduce animal dander:

– Keep your pet outside of the house or at least out of your bedroom.
– At least once a week, clean birdcages, rodent cages, or areas where pets sleep. Also, bathe your dog or cat on a weekly basis using veterinarian recommended shampoo.
– Dust and vacuum often. If you can, do this when the person who has an allergy or asthma is not at home. Use a static cloth for dusting, and use a vacuum with a high-efficiency particulate air (HEPA) filter, which helps keep dust off carpets and floors and out of the air.
– Keep air registers closed to reduce the amount of animal dander moving through the house.
– Do not allow your pet on carpets or upholstered furniture.
– Wash regularly any rugs, pillows, pet beds, or other items the pet has contacted.

If your symptoms are severe, it may be necessary to consider a new home for your pet.

• Mouse allergen exposure can be reduced by a combination of blocking access, low-toxicity pesticides, traps, and vacuuming and cleaning.
• House-dust mites:

Recommended steps:
- Encase mattress in an allergen-impermeable cover. Encase pillow in an allergen-impermeable cover or wash it weekly.
- Wash sheets and blankets on the patient's bed in hot water weekly (water temperature of >130°F is necessary for killing mites): cooler water and detergent and bleach will still reduce live mites and allergen level. Prolonged exposure to dry heat or freezing can also kill mites but does not remove allergen.
- Desirable: Reduce indoor humidity to or below 60%, ideally 30–50%; remove carpets from the bedroom; avoid sleeping or lying on upholstered furniture; remove carpets that are laid on concrete.
- Room air-filtering devices are not recommended for control of mite allergens because the allergens are associated with large particles which remain airborne for only a few minutes after disturbance. They are, therefore, not susceptible to removal by air filtration.
- Cockroaches:
  - Store food in airtight containers.
  - Clean all dirty dishes immediately after meals.
  - Clean up any food crumbs from the counters, stove top, tables, and floor.
  - Cover all trash cans tightly.
  - Avoid leaving pet food out in a bowl.
  - Fix leaky pipes under sinks and in the basement.
  - Seal cracks in the walls and floors.
  - Use cockroach baits and traps, but don't use sprays. Be careful to follow instructions on use, particularly in the kitchen.
- Pollens (from trees, grass, or weeds) and outdoor molds: If possible, adults who have allergies should stay indoors, with windows closed, during periods of peak pollen exposure, which are usually during the midday and afternoon.
- Indoor mold: Fix all leaks and eliminate water sources associated with mold growth; clean moldy surfaces. Consider reducing indoor humidity to or below 60%, ideally 30–50%. Dehumidify basements if possible.
- Air conditioning during warm weather, if possible, for patients who have asthma and are allergic to outdoor

allergens, because air conditioning allows windows and doors to stay closed, thus preventing entry of outdoor allergens. Regular use of central air conditioning also will usually control humidity sufficiently to reduce house-dust mite growth during periods of high humidity. Reducing relative humidity is a practical way to control house-dust mites and their allergens in homes in temperate climates.

- Formaldehyde and volatile organic compounds—which can arise from sources such as new linoleum flooring, synthetic carpeting, particleboard, wall coverings, furniture, and recent painting—have been implicated as potential risk factors for the onset of asthma and wheezing.
- Allergen immunotherapy should be considered for patients who have asthma if evidence is clear of a relationship between symptoms and exposure to an allergen to which the patient is sensitive. Controlled studies, usually conducted with single allergens, have demonstrated reduction in asthma symptoms caused by exposure to grass, cat, house-dust mite, ragweed, and two mold species.

Tobacco smoke

Patients and others in the home who smoke should stop smoking or smoke outside the home. Consider ways to reduce exposure to other sources of tobacco smoke, such as from daycare providers and the workplace.

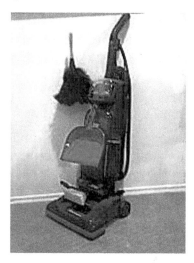

◀ Figure 16.3
Cleaning carpet with vacuum
Credit: Chuck Marean
Creative Commons

Indoor/Outdoor Pollutants and Irritants

Consider ways to reduce exposures to the following:
- Wood-burning stoves or fireplaces
- Unvented gas stoves or heaters
- Other irritants (e.g., perfumes, cleaning agents, sprays)
- Volatile organic compounds (VOCs) such as new carpeting, particle board, painting

Frequent house cleaning is very important to remove dust and pet dander that may contain allergens.

CHAPTER 17 *Special aspects of asthma in children*

106. Why is diagnosis of asthma difficult in children?

Young children, in particular, may have difficulty in describing symptoms to parents and physicians. It is usually not possible to conduct pulmonary function tests with very young children (0–4 years of age) because they may not be able to follow the instructions necessary to conduct the tests. The parents play an essential role in observing their child's symptoms. Parents should be able to describe the frequency and timing of symptoms, and whether they are associated with colds, and whether coughing or wheezing occur at other times.

The main symptoms of asthma in children are as follows:
- Wheeze
- Cough—when present with wheeze increases the likelihood of asthma
- Difficulty breathing
- Chest tightness

Asthma in early childhood is frequently underdiagnosed, resulting in many infants and young children not receiving adequate therapy. On the other hand, not all wheeze and cough are caused by asthma, and caution is needed to avoid giving infants and young children inappropriate prolonged asthma therapy.

Although wheezing is a prominent symptom of asthma, it may be due to other causes, including:

- Infections
  - Bronchiolitis-infection of the bronchioles, usually occurring in children less than 2 years old, due to a virus infection (respiratory syncytial virus).
  - Bronchitis — (also known as croup) affects the larynx or trachea and is typically worse at night.
- Reactive airways disease — a group of conditions that include reversible airway narrowing due to external stimulation. These conditions result in wheezing. The term sometimes is misused as a synonym for asthma. Current medical use of the term reactive airway disease is used in pediatrics to describe an asthma-like syndrome in infants that may later be confirmed to be asthmatics when they become old enough to participate in diagnostic tests such as the bronchial challenge test.
- Anatomic abnormalities
  - Adenoid hypertrophy — An enlargement of the adenoids which is very common in infants and preschool children. Symptoms include postnasal drip, snoring, and cough, especially at night.
  - Vocal cord dysfunction typically affects adolescents and young adults.
  - Tracheo-bronchomalacia — A condition in which cartilage rings in the trachea and/or bronchi are not rigid, resulting in retention of secretions, noisy breathing, and a tendency to infection.
- Foreign body aspiration — most common in the 1–3 year age group.
- GERD — Very common in young infants. Aspiration of gastric contents into the young can cause wheezing, and occasionally pneumonia.
- Congenital heart disease.
- Cystic fibrosis.

108. What should I consider as my asthmatic child attends school?

Most schools and daycare centers have many students with asthma, and may have developed asthma management programs.

These programs can include:
- A confidential list of students who have asthma.
- School policies and procedures for administering medications, including protocols for emergency response to a severe asthma episode.
- Specific actions for staff members to perform in the asthma management program.
- A written action plan for every student with asthma.
- Education for staff and students about asthma.

Schools should request that parents or guardians send a written student asthma action plan to school. This action plan should include daily management guidelines and emergency steps in case of an asthma episode. The plan should describe the student's medical information and specific steps for responding to worsening asthma symptoms. The asthma action plan should contain:
- A list of medications the student receives, noting which ones need to be taken during school hours. Also, medications needed during school activities "off-site" and "off-hours" should be noted and available.
- The plan should discuss if your child will be able to carry and self-administer his or her self-inhalers and other lifesaving medications at school. This self-administration will be dependent on if your doctor believes your child has the age, maturity, and developmental level for self-medication.
- A specific plan of action for school staff in case of an acute episode that includes guidance for monitoring peak flow.
- Identified triggers that can make asthma worse.
- Emergency procedures and phone numbers.

The action plan should be developed by a licensed health care provider or physician, signed by a parent and the physician, kept on file at school, and renewed every year. Because every student's asthma is different, the action plan must be specific to each student's needs.

The NAEPP has provided recommendations to schools to keep the environment clear of asthma-provoking substances. These include:

- Work with maintenance staff and environmental health specialists to set and monitor standards for school maintenance, humidity, ventilation and indoor air quality, mold, and dust control. Design and schedule building repairs, renovations, or cleaning to avoid exposing students and staff to fumes, dust, and other irritants. When possible, try to schedule painting and major repairs during long vacations or the summer months.
- Enforce smoking bans on school property.

The following steps should be taken with the school's physical education instructor and coach to encourage exercise and participation in sports for students with asthma:

- Be sure that the student's medications are available for exercise activities that take place away from school or after regular school hours. This preventive medicine enables most students with exercise-induced asthma to participate in any sport they choose.
- Warm-up and cool-down activities appropriate for any exercise will also help the student with asthma.
- Keep students' quick relief medications readily available. Even with precautions, breathing problems may occur. Learn the signs of severe distress and allergic reactions. Have an emergency plan. Don't delay getting medical help for a student with severe or persistent breathing difficulty.
- Encourage students with asthma to participate actively in sports, but also recognize and respect their limits. Plan to adjust the type, pace, or intensity of activities during extreme weather, the pollen season, poor air quality, or when a student has allergy symptoms or a peak flow number lower than usual. Be aware of the possibility of EIB if the sport takes place in cold, dry air. Permit less strenuous activities if a recent illness precludes full participation.

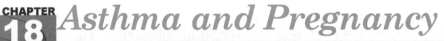

CHAPTER 18

Asthma and Pregnancy

109. What are the effects of pregnancy on my asthma?

- Pregnancy has variable effects on a woman's asthma: one-third of pregnant women improve, one-third worsen, and one-third experience no change in their condition. Women with severe asthma are more likely to worsen, while those with mild asthma are more likely to improve or remain unchanged.
- The change in the course of asthma in an individual woman during pregnancy tends to be similar in successive pregnancies.
- Asthma exacerbations are most likely to appear during the weeks 24–36 of gestation, with only occasional patients showing symptoms during labor and delivery.
- The changes in asthma noted during pregnancy usually return to pre-pregnancy status within 3 months of delivery.

There are a variety of theories regarding the worsening and improvement of asthma during pregnancy. For example, changes in chest wall conformation, an increased incidence of GERD, possible increased incidence of upper respiratory infections, and altered transfer of respiratory gasses in the lungs have been speculated to affect asthma during pregnancy.

110. What are the effects of hormonal changes during pregnancy on asthma?

Pregnancy results in an increase in the hormone estrogen producing an increased red cell mass. This change contributes to congestion of the capillaries (tiny blood vessels) in the lining of the nose, which in turn leads to a "stuffy" nose in pregnancy (especially during the third trimester). A rise in progesterone stimulates the respiratory center, and a feeling of shortness of breath may be experienced as a result of this hormonal increase. The respiratory system changes can lead to alterations in lung function measurements.

111. What are the dangers of uncontrolled asthma during pregnancy on the mother and fetus?

- Uncontrolled asthma causes a decrease in the mother's oxygen which, in turn, reduces the oxygen available to the developing fetus. This may result in impaired fetal growth; it could even affect survival of the fetus.

For a video on the effects of pregnancy on asthma, visit: http://acaai.org/asthma/who-has-asthma/pregnancy

ON THE WEB

- Dangerous blood pressure changes in the mother (known as preeclampsia).
- Premature birth.
- Increased emergency department visits.

112. What asthma medications are suitable during pregnancy?

- Inhaled medications are preferred because they have a more localized effect with only small amounts entering the bloodstream.
- Medication use should be limited in the first trimester as much as possible when the fetus is forming, even though birth defects from medications are rare.
- In general, the same medications used during pregnancy are appropriate during labor and delivery and when nursing. It is safer for pregnant women to be treated with asthma medications than for them to have asthma symptoms and exacerbations.

The National Asthma Education and Prevention Program (NAEPP) conducted a systematic review by drug class of the evidence on the safety of asthma medications during pregnancy. Regarding inhaled corticosteroids, the review found that "no studies to date have related inhaled corticosteroids to any increases in congenital malformations or other adverse perinatal outcomes."

NOTE

Perinatal pertains to or occurs in the period shortly before or after birth, variously defined as beginning with the completion of the twentieth to twenty-eighth week of gestation and ending 28 days after birth.

Likewise, the review found that beta$_2$-agonists and theophylline were safe when used at recommended doses. About oral (systemic) corticosteroids, the findings were conflicting. However, some studies showed that oral corticosteroid use was associated with an increased incidence of preeclampsia and the delivery of both preterm and low birth weight infants. Insufficient studies were available to evaluate the safety of leukotriene modifiers.

In preparing recommendations for treatment medications for asthma during pregnancy, the NAEPP classified asthma according to steps or severity. The classifications are: mild intermittent, mild persistent, moderate persistent, and severe persistent.

The following is a summary of NAEPP's stepwise approach for managing asthma:

- Step 1: Mild Intermittent Asthma.
  Short-acting bronchodilators, particularly short-acting inhaled beta$_2$- agonists, are recommended as quick-relief medication for treating symptoms as needed in patients with intermittent asthma. Albuterol is the preferred short-acting inhaled beta$_2$-agonist because it has an excellent safety profile and the greatest amount of data related to safety during pregnancy of any currently available inhaled beta$_2$-agonist. Women's experience with these drugs is extensive, and no evidence has been found either of fetal injury from the use of short-acting inhaled beta$_2$-agonists or of contraindication during lactation.
- Step 2: Mild Persistent Asthma.
  The preferred treatment for long-term control medication in Step 2 is daily low-dose inhaled corticosteroid. This preference is based on the strong effectiveness data in non-pregnant women as well as effectiveness and safety data in pregnant women that show no increased risk of adverse perinatal outcomes. Budesonide is the preferred inhaled corticosteroid because more data are available on using budesonide in pregnant women than are available on other inhaled corticosteroids, and the data are reassuring. It is important to note that there are no data indicating that the other inhaled corticosteroid preparations are unsafe during pregnancy. Therefore, inhaled corticosteroids other than budesonide may be continued in patients who were well controlled by these agents before pregnancy, especially if it is thought that changing formulations may jeopardize asthma control. Cromolyn, leukotriene receptor antagonists, and theophylline are listed as alternative but not preferred therapies. Cromolyn has an excellent safety record, but it has limited effectiveness compared with inhaled corticosteroids. Leukotriene receptor antagonists

have shown modest improvements in children and non-pregnant adults with asthma, although inhaled corticosteroids show more favorable outcomes. Published data are minimal on using leukotriene receptor antagonists during pregnancy although safety data are reassuring. Thus, leukotriene receptor antagonists are an alternative but not preferred treatment for pregnant women whose asthma was successfully controlled with this medication before their pregnancy. Theophylline has demonstrated clinical effectiveness in some studies and has been used for years in pregnant women with asthma. It also, however, has the potential for serious toxicity resulting from the excessive dosing and/or select drug-drug interactions (e.g., with erythromycin). Using theophylline during pregnancy requires careful monitoring of the dose.

- Step 3: Moderate Persistent Asthma.
  Two preferred treatment options are noted: either a combination of low-dose inhaled corticosteroid or a long-acting inhaled beta$_2$-agonist, or increasing the dose of inhaled corticosteroid to the medium dose range. No data from studies during pregnancy clearly delineate that one option is recommended over the other.
  Studies show that adding long-acting inhaled beta$_2$-agonist to a low dose of inhaled corticosteroid provides greater asthma control than only increasing the dose of corticosteroid. Two long-acting inhaled beta$_2$-agonists are available—salmeterol and formoterol.

- Step 4: Severe Persistent Asthma.
  If additional medication is required after carefully assessing patient technique and adherence with using Step 3 medication, then the inhaled corticosteroid dose should be increased within the high-dose range, and the use of budesonide is preferred. If this is insufficient to manage asthma symptoms, then systemic corticosteroid should be added. While the use of oral corticosteroids during pregnancy poses some uncertain risk, severe uncontrolled asthma poses a definite risk to the mother and fetus.

Rhinitis and sinusitis are often associated with asthma, are frequently more troublesome during pregnancy, and may exacerbate coexisting asthma. If these conditions are present, appropriate treatment is an integral part of asthma management. The following are recommendations on the use of medications to treat nasal conditions:

Rhinitis

- Intranasal corticosteroids are the most effective medications for the management of allergic rhinitis and have a low risk of systemic effect when used at recommended doses. These medications are used as nasal sprays. Montelukast, a leukotriene receptor antagonist, can be used for the treatment of allergic rhinitis—but minimal data are available on the use of this medication during pregnancy.
- The early antihistamines, such as Benadryl, have the drawback of causing drowsiness. The current second-generation antihistamines of choice are loratadine (Claritin) or cetirizine (Zyrtec). Antihistamines are taken orally by tablet or liquid.
- If nasal decongestion is indicated in early pregnancy, an external nasal dilator, short-term topical oxymetazoline, or intranasal corticosteroid can be considered before use of oral decongestants. There may be a relationship between use of oral decongestants in early pregnancy and a rare birth defect, gastroschisis.

Sinusitis

Sinusitis can result as a complication of rhinitis or the common cold.

This can make asthma worse, especially at night. Treating the inflammation in the nose and decreasing the post-nasal drip can reduce cough and throat irritation. Sinusitis is often treated with a saline nasal wash or a steroid nasal spray. Non-steroidal anti-inflammatory drugs (NSAIDs) are also used. Chronic sinusitis is normally treated with an antibiotic.

Traveling with Asthma

CHAPTER 19

114. If you have asthma, how should you plan for your trip?

- Check your medications: Make sure that you take along more than enough of all of your medicines and always keep them available.
- Check your devices to assure they are working well. If you are traveling in a foreign country, check to make sure you can operate your devices. Some foreign countries have other than 110 volt electrical power. If so, you may need to take a small portable transformer. Likewise, if the electrical outlet takes a different plug, you will need to take an adaptor to fit over your device plug. You should be able to find these adaptors in stores.
- Prepare a list of your medical conditions, medications, prescribing physician, and medications. Take along your written asthma action plan.
- Check the medical care at your destination: If your current insurance does not cover you during the trip, consider taking out supplemental travel insurance. Know where the medical facilities and pharmacies are and what the procedures are if you become sick.
- Plan your diet: If you have food allergies, be certain that the food you will be eating does not contain allergic substances. Advise anyone who will be preparing your food what you are allergic to as far in advance as possible.
- To protect against dust mites, pack your own allergy-proof pillow or mattress casings.
- If you or someone in your family has food or insect sting allergy, be sure to bring your self-injectable epinephrine. These are allowed on airplanes.

115. What should you consider, depending on your mode of travel?

- Plane
  - Pet allergy: Ask if any passenger on the same flight has made reservations with a pet and if so, can you can be seated away from the animal.
  - Air quality: Although most airlines now ban smoking on board, some international flights still permit

smoking. If smoking is permitted on your flight, ask for a seat that is furthest from the smoking sections. If you need oxygen, find out if the airlines can provide it or if you need to bring along your own supply.

- Food allergy: Find out what meals and snacks will be served on the flight. Ask if you can order a special meal if necessary.
- Tell the flight attendants about your medical condition. Wipe down your armrests and tray tables. Keep airline pillows or blankets in their plastic wrap and do not use.
- Drink plenty of fluids to stay hydrated
- Cruise
  - Advise cruise operators of your asthmatic condition. When you fill out the application form, there may be a place to list medical conditions.
  - Find out what medical facilities are available on the ship.
- Car
  - Keep your car clean (particularly the upholstery) to reduce the chances that dust mites and molds will ruin your trip.
  - If renting a car, try to get a late-model non-smoking vehicle.

116. What will you do at your destination?

- Visiting family/friends. Ask yourself the following questions:
  - Do my hosts know of my food allergies or asthmatic condition?
  - Do they have pets that I'm allergic to?
  - Is anyone in the home a smoker?
  - Staying in a hotel or resort. Check for cleanliness of the room, being particularly aware of a musty smell that could indicate the presence of molds.
  - Ask for a non-smoking room
- Take special coverings for pillows and beds, if you can
- Camping
  - To operate your devices, consider using portable nebulizers or a power inverter that can be plugged into your car receptacle.

References

CHAPTER 13

1. National Heart, Lung, and Blood Institute. "Asthma Action Plan." NIH Publication No. 07-5251. April 2007.
   https://www.nhlbi.nih.gov/files/docs/public/lung/asthma_actplan.pdf

CHAPTER 14

2. Canadian Center for Occupational Health and Safety. "Asthma, work-related." Last updated-5/1/2017
   https://www.ccohs.ca/oshanswers/diseases/asthma.html

3. Medline Plus. *https://medlineplus.gov/ency/article/000110.htm*

4. National Heart, Lung, and Blood Institute. "Employers, Employees and Worksites: Work-related asthma is a bigger problem than you think." Last Updated February 2011

   https://www.nhlbi.nih.gov/health-pro/resources/lung/naci/audiences/work.htm

5. Occupational Safety and Health Administration. "Do you have Work-Related Asthma?" March 2014
   https://www.osha.gov/Publications/OSHA3707.pdf

6. Wikipedia.*https://en.wikipedia.org/wiki/Occupational_asthma*

7. Vandenplas,Oliver. "Specific inhalation challenge in the diagnosis of occupational asthma: consensus statement." Eur Respir J 2014; 43: 1573–1587

   https://www.ncbi.nlm.nih.gov/pubmed/24603815

8. American Academy of Allergy Asthma & Immunology. "Occupational asthma." (2017).
   https://www.aaaai.org/conditions-and-treatments/library/at-a-glance/occupational-asthma

9. Medline Plus. "Occupational asthma." U.S. National Library of Medicine. April 30, 2015.
   https://medlineplus.gov/ency/article/000110.htm

10. Wikipedia. "Occupational asthma." Dec. 7, 2016.
    https://en.wikipedia.org/wiki/Occupational_asthma

CHAPTER 15

11. American College of Allergy, Asthma & Immunology. "Exercise-induced bronchoconstriction."(2014).
    http://acaai.org/asthma/exercise-induced-asthma-eib

12. Garry, Joseph. "Exercise-induced asthma." *Medscape*. WebMD. (2016).
    http://emedicine.medscape.com/article/1938228-overview

13. Schiffman, George. "Exercise-induced asthma." *eMedicine Health*. WebMD. April 21, 2016.
    http://www.emedicinehealth.com/exercise-induced_asthma/article_em.htm

CHAPTER 16

14. Diette, Gregory, Meredith C McCormack, Nadia N Hansel, Patrick N Breysse, and Elizabeth C Matsui. "Environmental issues in managing asthma." *Respiratory Care.* 53, no.5(2008):602–617.
   https://www.ncbi.nlm.nih.gov/pmc/articles/PMC2396450/

15. Strachan, David. "The role of environmental factors in asthma." *British Medical Bulletin.* 56, no. 4 (2000): 865–882.
   http://bmb.oxfordjournals.org

16. New York State Dept. of Health. "Environmental asthma triggers." Bulletin 4955, Aug. 2006.
   https://www.health.ny.gov/publications/4955.pdf

CHAPTER 17

17. Medline Plus. "Asthma in children." U.S. National Library of Medicine. Feb. 23, 2017.
   https://medlineplus.gov/asthmainchildren.html.

18. National Asthma Education and Prevention Program. "Managing asthma: a guide for schools." U.S. Dept. of Education- Document 02-2650. (2003).
   https://www.nhlbi.nih.gov/files/docs/resources/lung/asth_sch.pdf.

CHAPTER 18

19. American College of Allergy Asthma & Immunology. "Pregnancy and asthma." (2014).
   http://acaai.org/asthma/who-has-asthma/pregnancy

20. National Asthma Education and Prevention Program. "Managing asthma during pregnancy: recommendations for pharmacologic treatment, update 2004."
   https://www.nhlbi.nih.gov/files/docs/astpreg_qr.pdf

21. Petrache, Irina and Catherine Sears. "Asthma in pregnancy." *eMedicine Health*, WebMD. May 10, 2016.
   http://www.emedicinehealth.com/asthma_in_pregnancy/article_em.htm

CHAPTER 19

22. Asthma and Allergy Foundation of America. "Traveling with asthma and allergies." (Sept. 2015).
   http://www.aafa.org/page/traveling-with-asthma-allergies.aspx

23. Cleveland Clinic. "Traveling with asthma and allergies." (March 15, 2016).
   http://my.clevelandclinic.org/health/articles/traveling-with-asthma

Index

National Asthma Education and Prevention Program (NAEPP), 68, 80, 94, 137, 140
National Institute of Allergy and Infectious Diseases, 38
Nebulizers, 91
Nitric oxide test, 61
Nucleotides, 9
Non-allergic asthma, 14, 15
  Difference between allergic and, 14
  Major irritants triggering, 15
  Medical condition for, 15
Nonasthmatic eosinophilic bronchitis (NAEB), 52
Non-celiac gluten sensitivity (NCGS), 26
Non-steroidal antiinflammatory drugs (NSAIDs), 29, 56, 143

O

Occupational asthma, 124–127
  How to treat, 126–127
    Work aggravated and occupational induced, 126
  Physicians determining symptoms of, 125
  Workers at risk, 124
Occupational Safety and Health Administration (OSHA), 124

P

Parainfluenza viruses, 24
Parasympathetic nerves, 7
Patient education in asthma care, 122–124
  Cost analysis studies, 122
  Written asthma action plans, 123–124
Prick/puncture test, 62
Pulmonary arteries, 7
Pulmonary embolism, 53
Pulmonary function tests, 57–61
  Bronchoprovocation challenge test, 60–61
  Flow volume loops, 59–60
  Forced expiratory volume (FEV), 58–59, 62

Forced Vital Capacity (FVC), 59
Peak flow meters, 60
Positive methacholine bronchoprovocation test, 61
Spirometry, 58
Pulmonary veins, 7

R

Regurgitation, 22
Respiratory system, 5
Respiratory viral infections, 22–24
Respiratory syncytial virus (RSV), 22
Rhinovirus, 22
Rhinitis, 19
  Allergic, 19, 20
  Infectious, 19
  Non-allergic, 19
  Nose bronchi involvement, 20
  Types of, 19

S

Samter's trial, 56–57
Sensitization, 39
Severe acute respiratory syndrome (SARS), 24
Short-acting bronchodilators, 74
Sinuses, 24
Sinusitis, 24
Sputum eosinophils test, 62
Stimulation, 7
  Never receptor, 7
  Sympathetic system, 7
Systemic corticosteroids, 99–100

T

Theophylline, 106
  Questions before prescribing, 106–107
Tiotropium bromide, 111
Trachea or windpipe, 6
Traveler's asthma, 143
  Planning for trip, 143
  Things to consider, 143–144
  Things to do at your destination, 144
Type 2 T helper (Th2) cells, 39

V

Valved holding chamber (VHC), 82,
    85, 86, 88
Vocal cord dysfunction (VCD), 52
Vocal cords, 6
Volatile organic compounds
    (VOCs), 134

W

White blood cells (lymphocytes), 36
   Antibodies, 37

    IgG, 37
    IgA, 37
    IgE, 37, 39
   Antigen presenting cells (APCs),
    36
   Chemokines, 36
   B-cells, 37
   T-cells, 37